Addiction Treatment

Michael Weaver, MD

Professor of Psychiatry, University of Texas
Health Science Center, Houston, Texas

Medical Director,
Center for Neurobehavioral Research on Addiction

Published by Carlat Publishing, LLC
PO Box 626, Newburyport, MA 01950

CARLAT PSYCHIATRY

Addiction Treatment

Michael Weaver, MD, DFASAM
Professor of psychiatry at the University of Texas Health Science Center
in Houston, Texas
Medical director of the Center for Neurobehavioral Research on Addiction

Published by Carlat Publishing, LLC
PO Box 626, Newburyport, MA 01950

Publisher and Editor-in-Chief: Daniel Carlat, MD
Executive Editor: Janice Jutras

This CME/CE activity is intended for psychiatrists, psychiatric nurses, psychologists, and other health care professionals with an interest in mental health. The Carlat CME Institute is accredited by the Accreditation Council for Continuing Medical Education to provide continuing medical education for physicians. Carlat CME Institute is approved by the American Psychological Association to sponsor continuing education for psychologists. Carlat CME Institute maintains responsibility for this program and its content. The American Board of Psychiatry and Neurology has reviewed Addiction Treatment and has approved this program as a comprehensive Self-Assessment and CME Program, which is mandated by ABMS as a necessary component of maintenance of certification. Carlat CME Institute designates this enduring material educational activity for a maximum of four (4) ABPN Maintenance of Certification credits and eight (8) *AMA PRA Category 1 Credits*™ or 8 CEs for psychologists. Physicians or psychologists should claim credit commensurate only with the extent of their participation in the activity. CME quizzes must be taken online at www.thecarlatreport.com or http://thecarlatcmeinstitute.com/self-assessment.

To order, visit www.thecarlatreport.com or call (866) 348-9279

ISBN #: 978-0-9975106-3-8
eISBN #: 978-0-9975106-4-5

2 3 4 5 6 7 8 9 10

TABLE OF CONTENTS

Introduction v

Acknowledgments vi

CHAPTER 1: How to Diagnose Substance Use Disorder 1

CHAPTER 2: Drug Testing 17

CHAPTER 3: Understanding Addiction Services 35

CHAPTER 4: Psychotherapy 47

CHAPTER 5: 12-Step Programs 63

CHAPTER 6: Dual Diagnosis 81

CHAPTER 7: Alcohol 93

CHAPTER 8: Sedatives 117

CHAPTER 9: Nicotine 129

CHAPTER 10: Cannabis 145

CHAPTER 11: Opioids 157

CHAPTER 12: Stimulants 185

CHAPTER 13: Designer Drugs 195

CHAPTER 14: Hallucinogens and Other Drugs 205

Appendix 217

Clinical Institute Withdrawal Assessment of
Alcohol Scale, Revised (CIWA-Ar) 217

Clinical Opiate Withdrawal Scale 221

Drug Use Questionnaire (DAST-10) 224

Fagerström Test for Nicotine Dependence 226

Recommended Reading. 228

References 229

Self-Test Answer Key 233

Index 235

INTRODUCTION

I became interested in treating addictions as a medical student, and eventually, after doing a residency in internal medicine, completed a fellowship in addiction medicine. I found that in treating substance abuse, I could make a remarkable and rapid difference in people's lives. Over the years, as we've developed new and more effective treatments, managing addiction is no longer the province of addiction specialists—nor should it be. General psychiatrists and primary care doctors can learn the basics of an effective approach to treatment, and can gain the immense satisfaction that comes with helping people make dramatic changes in their lives.

I've divided the book into two sections. In the first section, I teach you general skills applicable to any patient with a substance use problem. I share tips on efficiently screening for the use of different substances in the initial interview, as well as ascertaining the severity of the disorder. I teach you about the appropriate use of drug screens, including how to talk to your patients about problematic results. In addition, I give you some psychotherapy pointers that are especially applicable to a busy MD who may be able to budget no more than 20–30 minutes for patient follow-ups. I devote a whole chapter to 12-step programs because they are often misunderstood by both clinicians and patients. In the comorbidity chapter, I cover the common problem of patients who present with a non–substance use issue, but in whom you realize that an addiction may be contributing to the problem.

The second section is organized by specific substances of abuse. For each substance, I cover the essentials of what it is, how it works in the brain, and what sort of withdrawal symptoms are likely to occur. Then I discuss practical approaches to assessing the problem, followed by how to treat the patient. Treatments vary depending on the substance; sometimes they will be primarily psychosocial, other times mainly medication-based.

Finally, I've added various useful tools in the Appendix and have provided links to access these materials in the electronic version of this book.

ACKNOWLEDGMENTS

This is my opportunity as author to acknowledge and thank all the people without whom this book would not be possible. I owe many thanks to Danny Carlat and the entire Carlat Publishing team for all their invaluable help with this effort, and without whom there would be no book. I must thank my family, who allowed me to take time away from them to spend on writing this. I want to thank Sidney Schnoll, my mentor, for many years of encouragement and wise advice. Finally, I should thank Joan Peck, my nurse at the methadone clinic for many years, who told me countless times that I need to write a book—well, Joan, here it is.

CHAPTER 1

How to Diagnose Substance Use Disorder

"I used to think a drug addict was someone who lived on
the far edges of society. Wild-eyed, shaven-headed and
living in a filthy squat. That was until I became one . . ."
Cathryn Kemp, *Painkiller Addict: From Wreckage
to Redemption—My True Story*

TAKE HOME POINTS

- Dopamine desensitization underlies most substance abuse.
- During your first interview, ascertain what substances are being used, how they are negatively affecting the patient's life, and how motivated the patient is to change.
- Use normalization to decrease stigma.
- When asking about specific drugs, start with the most socially acceptable substances and end with the most stigmatizing.
- Use the DSM-5 mnemonic: Tempted With Cocaine, Scotch, Rum.

CASE VIGNETTE: *G is a 45-year-old woman who presents for treatment of anxiety. She was prescribed alprazolam (Xanax) by her family practitioner to take once or twice daily for severe anxiety symptoms, but she has been taking it closer to 3 times every day. She also has 2 drinks of gin before bedtime most nights, and has done this for several years. She tells me that occasionally she will get "shaky" during the day, and an alprazolam or a drink will steady her nerves.*

WHAT IS SUBSTANCE USE DISORDER?

Before diving into the skills of diagnosing substance use disorders, it's fair to take a step back and ask what a substance use disorder actually is. Is it a brain disease? Is it self-medication? Is it a life choice?

The answer can be any of the above, or a combination, depending on the person and the substance. For the opioid addict with overwhelming cravings who is stealing money from her friends to buy her next fix, it is primarily a brain disease involving opiate receptors. For the college student taking Adderall a couple of times a week—borrowed from friends—to study for exams and write papers, it may be a lifestyle choice (though it can devolve into neurochemical dependency if the habit becomes a daily one). For the man with social anxiety disorder who downs a few shots of vodka before going to a social event, it may be a form of self-medication.

Like most disorders in medicine and psychiatry, substance use is multifactorial, and for this same reason, it can be treated in different ways.

Neurobiology of addiction

While our knowledge of the neurobiology of addiction is limited, researchers are beginning to work out some of the mechanisms. One particular neurotransmitter, dopamine (DA), seems to play a central role for most addictions.

Most psychiatrists are familiar with DA in the setting of psychosis. All antipsychotics block DA receptors, which implies that excessive DA can be a bad thing, as it may be one of the chemicals that can cause psychosis.

However, there is another side of DA—it's the primary neurotransmitter for the brain's reward system. Our brain releases high levels of DA during joyful events, like graduating from high school, winning a race, or enjoying a Thanksgiving dinner. Another experience that can cause a kind of "joy" is abusing drugs. Cocaine and methamphetamine cause the most DA release, leading the user to feel intensely exhilarated and powerful.

While a large release of DA can indeed produce positive emotions, the brain quickly institutes measures to maintain a stable internal environment, or homeostasis. One measure is to quickly clear the DA away, which the brain does by breaking the DA down with enzymes or recycling it. But when someone is consistently using drugs, there's too much DA for this process to work. Therefore, the brain alters itself to make the neurons a little less receptive to DA. This process is called "desensitization," and it occurs in various ways biochemically, such as decreasing the number of DA receptors or slowing down receptor activation.

As the brain desensitizes to DA, the drug user experiences this as tolerance, meaning the person does not experience the same high from a given dose. If the dose is increased to compensate, the user will get high, but the brain will go through its homeostasis process again, forming tolerance to the higher dose. This is a simplistic neurobiological explanation of tolerance.

What about withdrawal—why does that happen? When there's no external stimulation causing the brain to release DA, the user must depend on the old-fashioned process of the brain releasing DA as it normally would: that is, in response to the prosaic pleasurable events of life, like having a snack or watching a ball game. But a brain that has gotten used to relying on high levels of DA has fewer DA receptors, and those receptors are less sensitive. Therefore, the normal amount of DA doesn't produce much, if any, pleasure compared to what the addict experiences when getting a "fix." When an addict's drug of choice is taken away, a DA deficiency results. This is one reason withdrawal is so unpleasant, and why stimulant withdrawal causes depression. With a damaged reward circuit, it becomes very hard for a user to experience normal healthy behaviors as motivating. The temptation to use drugs is extreme, because the user now feels the drugs are needed simply to feel normal. (For a review of the dopamine theory of addiction, see Nutt DJ et al, *Nature Reviews Neuroscience* 2015;16:305–312.)

Genetics of addiction

Drug addiction often runs in families, though the strength of the development of addiction varies between substances. Familial transmission of substance abuse does not necessarily imply genetic involvement; however, there is in fact a large amount of evidence that genes play a role.

One piece of evidence comes from studies of identical and fraternal twins. The most interesting of these studies compares these two types of twins when they have been separated at birth and put up for adoption. If addiction had nothing to do with genes, but everything to do with upbringing, one might expect that the diagnostic concordance rate of identical and fraternal twins would be the same—but in fact the identical twin concordance rate is higher. Using this kind of data, studies have estimated that the heritability of addiction to alcohol and drugs in general is 60%. This does not mean that a patient has a 60% chance of developing an addiction if one of the patient's parents had an addiction, although this is a common misunderstanding. Instead, if a person becomes addicted, about 60% of the reason for that addiction will be genetic, while about 40% of it will be non-genetic—such as the effects of upbringing (Yu & McClellan, 2016).

If genetics has so much to do with addiction, what are some of the possible genes that play a part, and how might they work? A number of genetic variants have been identified that might contribute to increasing a person's vulnerability to addiction. For example, genes for certain sub-types of GABA-A receptors have an association with alcohol use disorder, and a different cluster of genes is associated with a higher risk for nicotine use disorder. Other gene variants can protect against addiction. In several Asian populations, gene variants for alcohol dehydrogenase cause disulfiram-like reactions, making drinking very unpleasant. Overall, however, we're still quite far from truly understanding the genetics of addiction, and there is no clinically useful genetic test for helping us predict who is likely to become addicted.

CASE REVISITED: *When I ask about problems that run in her family, G reveals that her father was an alcoholic, just like his father had been. She also admits that her son has been using cannabis heavily, and that she and her husband sent him to an addiction treatment program a couple of years ago when he was in his late teens. This was a very stressful experience for her.*

ASSESSMENT OF SUBSTANCE USE DISORDER
Purpose of the evaluation

When you are evaluating patients for addiction, it's helpful to keep in mind these three common types of patients:

1. *The treatment seeker.* This patient comes to you explicitly for substance use treatment, and is willing to lay all the cards on the table to get better. The evaluation will be straightforward and aimed at ascertaining information to build the best treatment plan.

2. *The treatment willing.* This patient comes to you for a psychiatric issue, and is also abusing substances. However, the patient doesn't consider the substance abuse a problem—not because of denial but more because of

ignorance about the potential mental health effects. You will have to work a little bit harder to get the patient's substance history, but it won't be too difficult, because the person is not trying to hide anything from you.

3. *The hider.* This patient is willfully abusing substances and wants to continue doing so. The person may come to you for treatment of a separate psychiatric issue, or might just be in your office to score some scheduled drugs. Hiders are difficult patients and require the most skill and intuition for a good evaluation.

The questions you ask and the approach you take will differ depending on the type of patient you suspect you are dealing with. In all cases, you'll want to obtain the following information:

- What substances is the patient using, how much, and how often?
- How is the substance use negatively affecting different aspects of the patient's life? How severe is the problem? The severity informs lots of treatment decisions, such as how difficult detoxification will be, whether detox should occur in the inpatient or outpatient setting, and what kinds of referrals for adjunctive treatment you should be making.
- How motivated is the patient to decrease or discontinue drug use? Does the patient believe there is a problem? This is crucial because a big part of treatment is harnessing and increasing the patient's internal motivation to get on track to a substance-free life. You need to find out "where the person is" in terms of desire for treatment.
- What type of treatment has the patient had in the past, and what helped? Through what is called treatment matching, you'll try to match the severity of the disorder with the least restrictive treatment environment that is likely to be effective. For example, someone with no psychosocial support and a lot of physical withdrawal symptoms would probably not be a great fit for outpatient treatment. In contrast, if you have a patient with a supportive family and low levels of physical tolerance, then individual outpatient counseling may be a good option.

Screening questions: General tips

At some point in your initial psychiatric interview, you should plan to do a thorough screen for drug use. The launching point for that screen will vary. It might be during the first few minutes, while the patient is giving an introduction and explaining the reason for the appointment. If drug use figures prominently in the initial history of your patient's present illness, you can start your substance screening then. Alternatively, if you typically ask about health habits, like smoking or drinking coffee, you could start the screening questions there. You can also make the transition less organic and simply plan to talk about it a bit later in the interview, once you've had a chance to build rapport.

Before diving into the specifics of particular substances, however, it's important to recognize that substance use questions are tough to ask—and for patients to answer. People are embarrassed to admit to using drugs, partly because they worry others will see it as a personal weakness or defect. In that sense, it's not much different from the stigma that accompanies any psychiatric disorder. But substance use carries legal ramifications as well. People are concerned about being arrested or about losing jobs, child custody, or driving privileges, among other things.

For all these reasons, you should be sensitive in broaching this subject. My approach is to try to normalize substance use as much as possible. I want to reassure the patient that I consider substance use a common behavior—one that is defensible and sometimes almost expected in some situations. Here are some tips on introducing the topic of substance abuse:

If the patient is describing depressive symptoms, I might say, "Different people get relief from symptoms in different ways. What sorts of things have you tried for your depression?" Patients will usually tell me that they've taken antidepressants, had therapy, or used some type of self-help strategy. I'll follow that up with, "Some people have found relief in other ways, such as using marijuana to help calm down or lifting their mood by using a stimulant or alcohol. Have you tried something like that and found it to be helpful, or not helpful?" This gives patients permission to describe some non-mainstream approaches they may have taken. I might also say, "Some people taking a prescription medication for one reason find that it helps with their mood or with other symptoms. Have you ever noticed anything like this?"

If you're transitioning to the drug screen part of an appointment, one way to make the transition is to say, "I'm going to ask questions about different drugs you may have used." Asking about substances is not just for the initial evaluation, of course. If you've been seeing a patient for a while and there hasn't been the kind of progress you would expect, you might suspect that substance use is playing a part. You can ask, "How often over the past month have you gotten a buzz?" Explain to the patient that drug or alcohol use might be interfering with progress in terms of symptom management.

Screening questions for specific substances

I recommend starting with the more socially accepted drugs and gradually working your way to the more stigmatizing. I often start with smoking because it's socially accepted. Here are some sample questions that you may want to use based on substance type:

Nicotine

This one is simple: "Do you smoke?" If patients say yes, I'll ask when they started, how much they use, and so forth. If they say no, I'll follow up with, "Have you ever smoked?" and, "When did you last smoke?" Surprisingly, some people who consider themselves nonsmokers will respond with, "I last smoked two days ago." While they may believe they are out of the woods because of a very recent quit attempt, we know that relapse rates are high, and this is important information to gather.

Caffeine

You can introduce the topic of caffeine by saying, "Let me get an idea of your health habits. Do you drink coffee, tea, or soda?" If patients say "no," that's quite unusual, and I'll want to know why, because usually it's a health reason; if so, I praise them for a good health decision. After asking about typical caffeinated beverages, I move on to energy drinks, which can be stigmatizing: "Do you drink any energy drinks, like Red Bull, AMP, or Monster?" Using the names of the beverages helps to establish your "street cred" before you move on to discuss more serious substances. Just referring to them as "energy drinks" may make your patients feel less connected with you and less forthcoming with the truth; they may even not know exactly what you are asking about.

Alcohol

Given that alcohol is socially acceptable and widely used, I preface my screening question with a normalizing comment: "Most people drink. How much do you drink in terms of beer, wine, or whiskey?" I don't start by using the term "alcohol" because some people think about drinking alcohol in terms of an alcoholic drinking from a whiskey bottle in a paper bag. If they have a couple of beers a night or a nightcap before bedtime, they may not see that as drinking alcohol.

Prescription and over-the-counter meds

I ask questions like, "What sort of meds that don't require a prescription have you taken, like Robitussin or Sudafed?" "Have you taken them in ways other than the directions on the package?" "What about prescription medications? Have you taken them in ways that are different from how they were prescribed?" Since taking extra prescription drugs is stigmatizing, I'll give patients implicit permission by adding, "Folks may find that it's more helpful for them to take more medications than are prescribed."

Cannabis

Since medical marijuana and recreational use of cannabis products is becoming legal in more states, patients are more likely to be open about their cannabis use, even if you are in a state that hasn't legalized it. Asking about cannabis is a good segue from legal to illegal drug use. You can ask, "Most people have tried marijuana at some point in their lives; when have you tried it?" A lot of people will say, "When I was a teen." If so, you can follow up by asking whether they were regular users, and whether they aged out of it.

⬤ **CLINICAL PEARL:**
What Is "Experimentation"?

One way of asking about drug use in a less threatening way is to couch it in terms of experimentation, as in, "Have you ever experimented with marijuana or LSD?" But what does the term "experimentation" really mean? In terms of substance use diagnoses, we consider 6 or fewer uses to be experimentation, whereas more than 6 uses rises to the level of diagnosis of a DSM substance use disorder.

At this point in the screening interview, you've asked about many substances, and the patient should realize you are not passing judgment. This will let you more comfortably ask, in a matter-of-fact way, about illegal substances. Often, rather than going through each illegal substance, I ask, "What other kinds of drugs have you used?" or, "Is there something you've used that I haven't asked about?" If the patient doesn't seem forthcoming, I'll run through the classes of drugs.

Stimulants

If a patient has been prescribed stimulant medications for attention deficit hyperactivity disorder, I will ask about misuse of those medications, or ask whether the patient has taken prescription stimulants without a prescription: "Have you ever used Adderall or Ritalin to study for a test or finish a project on time?" This provides a specific reason that the patient can affirm, which is less stigmatizing. It can also help with the transition to asking about illicit stimulants, which can have similar effects to prescribed stimulants: "Have you used things like cocaine or amphetamines, sometimes known as snow, ice, coke, or speed?" Similar to naming energy drinks, asking in this way establishes street cred and provides an opportunity to give the patient examples.

Opioids

You can ask, "Lots of people have taken prescription painkillers in ways that aren't prescribed; is that something you've tried?" Give specific examples like Percocet, OxyContin, Vicodin, and others. This not only encourages honesty, but also may give you useful information about whether patients know what drug they have been taking. The reality is that some people may buy an opioid on the street and have no idea what it is—only that their dealer says it's good. You can also ask, "Have you used heroin, dope, or smack?"

Hallucinogens

You can ask, "A lot of people have tried things like LSD or mushrooms or acid. What's been your experience?"

Inhalants

Questions about inhalants include, "Have you ever huffed or sniffed something?" or, "Have you used things like poppers, or laughing gas, or household products like spray paint, hair spray, whipped cream, paint thinner, or airplane glue to get high?"

Designer drugs

For designer drugs, you can ask, "Have you tried synthetic marijuana or bath salts?" or, "Have you tried any club drugs like ecstasy or special K?"

CASE REVISITED: *G describes significant use of alcohol in addition to her prescribed use of alprazolam. I perform a quick screen for other substances.*

I do not go through every single drug, as I sense that she is being forthcoming in her responses.

Doctor: Most people have tried marijuana at some point in their lives. When have you done that?

G: Oh, it's been a long time since I've used that.

Doctor: A lot of people use it in high school, often with their friends. Was that how you got started?

G: Yes, I smoked it with my friends after school and at parties.

Doctor: How long after high school did you continue to smoke marijuana regularly?

G: Oh, for a few years, but I stopped after I got married.

Doctor: Did you try any other drugs with your friends in high school?

G: Yes. I tried magic mushrooms a couple of times, but I never got into that or any other drugs.

Doctor: So, you smoked some weed regularly with your friends in high school and after that until you got married, and you tried mushrooms a couple of times. How about other drugs you tried?

G: No, nothing else. I was too afraid to ever try anything like heroin or cocaine.

I am reassured that the only substances G is overusing are alprazolam and alcohol. Subsequent random drug screens confirm that she is being truthful.

DSM-5: CRITERIA FOR SUBSTANCE USE DISORDER

DSM-5 made life easier for those of us who see patients with substance use disorders. Under DSM-IV, we had to remember two ways of describing substance problems: substance dependence vs. substance abuse. Distinguishing these two was neither easy nor particularly meaningful in terms of treatment decisions.

In DSM-5, the criteria for dependence and abuse have been combined into one long list of 11 criteria. Depending on how many criteria patients meet, they are diagnosed with mild, moderate, or severe substance use disorder. Here's the breakdown for severity:

- Mild: 2–3 criteria
- Moderate: 4–5 criteria
- Severe: 6 or more criteria

As was true for DSM-IV, the criteria are almost exactly the same for all substances, so once you memorize the basic list, you've memorized it for all substances. The exceptions to this are:

- There is no caffeine use disorder, but there are DSM-5 diagnoses for caffeine intoxication and caffeine withdrawal.
- Some classes of drugs do not have withdrawal symptoms that have been clearly established in humans, so the withdrawal criterion is not included in the diagnosis. These drug classes are:
  —Hallucinogens (an exception to this exception is MDMA, which does have a withdrawal syndrome similar to other stimulants because it is chemically related to stimulants)
  —Phencyclidine
  —Inhalants

While you might have the DSM-5 on your desk or on your smartphone, you can also memorize the criteria by using the mnemonic below.

Mnemonic for DSM-5 substance use disorder:

Tempted **W**ith **C**ocaine, **S**cotch, **R**um
(**T**olerance, **W**ithdrawal, **C**ontrol, **S**ocial, **R**isky)

The patient must meet at least 2 of the following 11 criteria within a 12-month period:
  1. **T**olerance, that is, a need for increasing amounts of substance to achieve intoxication
  2. **W**ithdrawal syndrome

Loss of **C**ontrol *of substance use (4 criteria):*
  3. Cravings
  4. Using more than planned
  5. Unable to quit despite attempts to do so
  6. Much time spent obtaining or recovering from substance

Social consequences (3 criteria):
  7. Important social, occupational, or recreational activities given up or reduced because of substance use

8. Failure to fulfill major role obligations at work, school, or home

9. Persistent social and interpersonal problems caused by substance

Risky use (2 criteria):

10. Continued substance use despite the patient's knowledge of significant physical or psychological problems caused by its use

11. Recurrent substance use in physically hazardous situations

If you're confused about the differences between DSM-IV and DSM-5 criteria for substance use disorder, here is a graphic that might be useful (Figure 1-1).

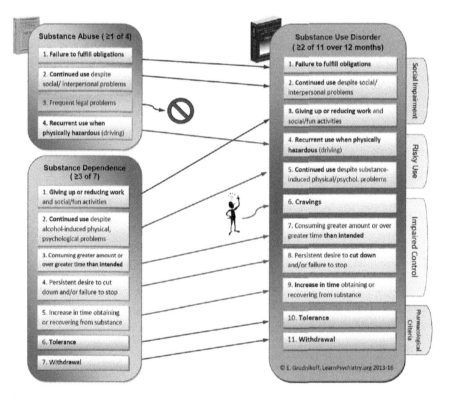

FIGURE 1-1. DSM-IV vs. DSM-5 Substance Use Disorder Criteria
(Illustration courtesy of Eugene Grudnikoff, from his website, learnpsychiatry.org. http://learnpsychiatry.org/w/index.php?title=File:Substance_use_project.JPG)

Ascertaining DSM criteria

In the screening portion of the interview, you determined which substances the patient has used. Now what? Going through each of the 11 DSM criteria in turn could get rather tedious. Instead, I recommend getting at the criteria as organically as possible by asking open-ended questions during the evaluation. For example:

- "What kinds of problems has your use of these drugs caused for you?"
- "Have there been any drawbacks to using that drug?"
- "It seems like you are handling some things pretty well. Are there other things that are concerning for you?"
- "Tell me about any problems you have had at home or work."

From experience, I have a good sense of the consequences—emotional, financial, family, career, etc—of substance abuse. As patients talk about what they are using, I assess the life areas that have most likely been impacted by their substance use. If they don't talk much, I'll get more specific in my questions, and I might then use a checklist to fill in gaps.

CASE REVISITED: *What is G's diagnosis? Here are a few of the questions I ask her during our session:*

Doctor: What kinds of problems has your use of these drugs caused for you?

G: Well, I take the Xanax for my anxiety, but it wears off too quick.

Doctor: That means you have tolerance to that drug. The worsening anxiety you feel may be an early withdrawal symptom. This may also be happening when you feel "shaky" during the day sometimes and take something to calm your nerves. Have you had to take more than you planned to?

G: Yes.

Doctor: Any other problems?

G: Sometimes I get anxious about the amount of housework I have to get done, so I take a Xanax to settle my nerves, but then I'm not able to get the housework done after all.

Doctor: So you have trouble fulfilling some of your obligations at home.

G: That's right.

With just a few questions, I have demonstrated DSM criteria related to tolerance and withdrawal, loss of control, and social consequences. I establish a diagnosis of moderate sedative use disorder.

Surveys/screening tools

Are surveys and screening tools useful for a psychiatrist? They can be, especially if you have patients fill them out in the waiting room before the appointment. You can then both go over the answers as a way of making sure nothing gets missed and saving time otherwise spent in asking a series of questions.

While there are many substance-related questionnaires available, here are two that are brief enough to be practical for a general psychiatrist. Both are free and available online (see Appendix).

- PHQ, the Patient Health Questionnaire, screens for depression, anxiety, eating disorders, and alcohol use. It can be broken down into individual modules or given as one longer instrument for the patient to complete. (http://www.phqscreeners.com/)
- DAST, the Drug Abuse Screening Test, is a 10-item questionnaire that screens for problematic drug use. (https://cde.drugabuse.gov/instrument/e9053390-ee9c-9140-e040-bb89ad433d69)

CASE CONCLUSION: *After gathering information from G about her current problems with prescription medications and alcohol, as well as her family history of addiction and other drugs she has tried previously, I ask about current (within the past 12 months) problems related to drug and alcohol use. This information allows me to make a diagnosis of sedative use disorder, moderate, and alcohol use disorder, mild. When I summarize this information for G and inform her that it has led me to specific substance use disorder diagnoses, it helps her understand that her problems are directly related to how she is using Xanax and alcohol. Now she is more willing to consider making changes in her behavior.*

Self-Test Questions

1. Which of the following substances does not have a formal substance use disorder, according to the DSM-5?
   a. Caffeine
   b. Tobacco
   c. Cannabis
   d. Phencyclidine

2. A high school student is learning about genetics in his science class. When he was 10 months old, he was adopted by parents who did not drink alcohol or use illicit drugs. He recently learned that his biological parents drank alcohol heavily and used illicit drugs, which is why he was removed from that home and later adopted. The percentage of his risk for developing a substance use disorder that is due to genetic heritability is:
   a. 0%
   b. 10%
   c. 33%
   d. 60%

3. You are seeing a 65-year-old male patient for evaluation of depression. You verify that he has no health problems besides mild hip and back pain from osteoarthritis. When asked, the patient tells you he drinks 2 beers every evening. Once in a while on a weekend he will have a few more beers, usually without initially intending to do so. He drinks at home, so he has never driven while drunk, and his wife has never seemed concerned about his drinking. The patient admits that he has thought his drinking may not be helping his depression, but he has no desire to cut back despite this. Based on this information, this patient has which of the following diagnoses?
   a. Alcohol use disorder, mild
   b. Alcohol use disorder, moderate
   c. Alcohol use disorder, severe
   d. Alcohol use disorder in sustained remission

The answer key for these self-test questions is on page 233.

Note: If you purchased CME credit with this book, your CME post-test can be accessed when you are logged in at www.thecarlatreport.com/AddictionGuide. Please keep in mind that the question and answer order for that CME post-test are different than what you see in these self-test study questions.

CHAPTER 2

Drug Testing

"Why is there so much controversy about drug testing? I know plenty of guys who would be willing to test any drug they could come up with."
George Carlin

TAKE HOME POINTS

- Order drug screens for patients who have a history of drug use or who have a psychiatric disorder that is not responding well to standard treatments.
- A urine drug screen is the most common and appropriate test for most patients.
- Actual false positive results are extremely rare.
- Order confirmatory testing if there is uncertainty about the meaning of a test result.
- Use positive results as opportunities to improve your treatment program and to enhance your alliance with your patient.

CASE VIGNETTE: *A 38-year-old man, D, presents to you with depression and a history of two hospitalizations for bipolar disorder. One discharge summary from several years ago mentions "alcohol abuse" as a discharge diagnosis. When you ask about this, D says this was a "misunderstanding" and maintains he's never been an alcoholic. As you go through your standard questions about substance abuse, D acknowledges having used many drugs when he was younger, but says "that's not a problem anymore." His medication list from his last provider includes lithium, bupropion, and lorazepam. He says he isn't taking the lithium, but that the lorazepam helps his anxiety.*

You are concerned about D's drug abuse history, and you would like to get a urine drug screen. However, you don't want to alienate him by implying that you doubt his claim about drugs no longer being a problem.

WHEN TO ORDER A DRUG SCREEN

You should order a drug screen for any patient who has a substance use disorder, or whom you suspect may have one. Drug screens are the key diagnostic tests that help us determine what we are treating and whether our treatment is successful. They are the only way to keep patients accountable for what they tell you, because substance-using patients are often ashamed of their use and hide the truth. Drug screening is not about "catching" or punishing patients. Instead, it's a way to help establish honesty and accountability.

At a minimum, you should order drug screens in the following situations:

- Your patient has a current or recent substance use problem. This is the major reason to get a drug screen: monitoring the sobriety of patients who are acknowledged drug/alcohol users and want to get clean.
- Your patient has a remote substance use problem and you are considering prescribing a medication with potential for abuse.
- Your patient is not improving despite receiving evidence-based treatment, and you are wondering if drug use is interfering with treatment. The estimated lifetime prevalence of drug or alcohol abuse in depression is 16%–27%, in bipolar disorder 43%–56%, and in schizophrenia 20%–65%, depending on the study methodology used (Bradizza et al, 2006). The lifetime prevalence of drug abuse in the general population is around 8% (Compton et al, 2007), and around 18% for alcohol abuse (Hasin et al, 2007).
- You are prescribing a controlled substance medication (such as a psychostimulant or a benzodiazepine) and your patient has been requesting early refills or increased dosages.

HOW TO BROACH THE ISSUE WITH PATIENTS

CASE REVISITED: *You decide that a urine drug screen is clearly indicated for D, for multiple reasons: He has a history of substance abuse, he is requesting a refill of lorazepam, and you are concerned about his lack of response to standard treatment for bipolar disorder.*

You tell D, "I'd like to order a urine drug screen along with a lithium level."

D responds defensively, saying, "Why would you order a urine drug screen?"

Broaching the topic of drug testing can be uncomfortable for both you and your patient. Patients often assume that drug screening is about "catching" their drug use, and fear that they will be punished in some way for it.

If you work in an addiction treatment clinic, you can frame drug testing as a standard procedure for all patients: "Like most programs, we do random urine drug testing. The reason for it is to provide an objective measure of what you've been using, which can help confirm that you are telling the truth."

The situation is trickier in a private practice setting, but you can take away some of the stigma by framing it as part of your typical routine: "It's part of my practice to get urine drug screens. I do this as a diagnostic test. I want to see what's in your system so I can better design a treatment plan for you." Share with patients that you know it may be hard for them to disclose what is in their system, and point out that it's possible something they are taking is interfering with their antidepressants and/or other medications. Assure them that testing is not done to catch them in the act of drug use—that's a job for a parole officer. The point is not to punish patients for a positive result; rather, it's an opportunity to intervene therapeutically.

I often use the analogy of building up good credit. I will say something like: "If you usually pay bills on time, you develop good credit, and then you make the occasional late payment, a business is likely to overlook that. Similarly, if I see that you have only an occasional urine sample with a problematic result, then that's more easily overlooked and less concerning than if it happens with increasing frequency."

In general, while drug testing can theoretically be a source of conflict, you might be surprised at how rarely it occurs. Sometimes patients are relieved that they don't have to tell us face-to-face what they've been using and that we have a straightforward test to get that information.

CASE REVISITED: *You respond to D's defensiveness by saying: "Here's why I'd like to do drug testing. You have bipolar disorder, and I've found that a lot of my patients with bipolar disorder don't realize that even small amounts of alcohol or drugs can interfere with treatment. Because of this, I always do drug testing so I can make sure our treatment is on the right track." D is amenable.*

WHICH TYPE OF SPECIMEN SHOULD YOU ORDER?

Specimens of urine, blood, hair, saliva, sweat, and even nails can be used to do lab drug testing. See Table 2-1 for more detail on types of drug tests. Most clinicians will order only urine testing.

TABLE 2-1. Available Drug Tests

Test	Detection Time Frame	Notes
Urine	3–4 days	Most commonly used
Blood	6–12 hours	Can detect only recent drug use
Hair	7 days–3 months	Expensive, but good for discovering use in more distant past
Saliva	24 hours	Convenient; patients can't adulterate or substitute; may not detect benzodiazepines
Sweat	7–14 days	Patient can remove patch
Nails	7 days–3 months	Not commonly ordered
Breathalyzer (for alcohol only)	A few hours	Often used by patient's family to assess driving safety

Urine

Urine drug testing is the most common test ordered because it's noninvasive, it's available in large volume, and it generally has high concentrations of drugs and metabolites (allowing for a longer detection time frame than in blood, for example). Many factors can affect how soon and for how long a drug can be detected, but you can make reasonable predictions. It takes about 2–3 hours for most drugs to be concentrated in urine (only 30 minutes for alcohol), so testing too soon after use in a non-chronic user of a drug may give you a negative result. Most drugs will be detected in urine for about 2–4 days after use; some will be detected for longer (see Table 2-2 for urine testing detection windows).

Although labs vary, there are two common urine drug screening panels that you can order: basic and comprehensive. The basic test screens for 5 drugs: amphetamines, cocaine, marijuana, some opiates, and phencyclidine. The comprehensive panel adds methadone (and sometimes other opiates) and sedative/hypnotic medications, such as benzodiazepines, barbiturates, and the "z-drugs" like zolpidem (Ambien) and zaleplon (Sonata).

TABLE 2-2. Urine Testing Detection Periods by Drug

Drug	Detection Period for Urine Testing
Alcohol	7–12 hours
Alcohol metabolites, ethyl glucuronide and ethyl sulfate (ETG/ETS)	3–4 days
Amphetamine/methamphetamine	1–2 days
Barbiturates	2–4 days (2–3 weeks for long-acting phenobarbital)
Benzodiazepines	24 hours (short-acting); 2–4 days (long-acting); > 7 days for chlordiazepoxide, diazepam
Cocaine	6–8 hours (2–4 days for benzoylecgonine metabolite)
LSD	2–4 days
Marijuana	3 days for single use; 5–7 days for moderate use (4x/week); 10–15 days for daily use; > 30 days for long-term heavy use
MDMA	1–2 days
Nicotine	12 hours
Opioids • Codeine • Buprenorphine • Heroin, hydromorphone, morphine, oxycodone • Methadone	 1–2 days 2–3 days (5–7 days metabolites) 2–4 days 2–3 days; 7–9 days for chronic use
PCP	2–8 days; up to 30 days for chronic use

Adapted from: Moeller KE et al, *Mayo Clin Proc* 2008;83(1):66–76.
Warner EA and Sharma N. Laboratory diagnosis. In Ries RK, Miller SC, Fiellen DA, Saitz R, eds. *Principles of Addiction Medicine*. 4th ed. Philadelphia: Lippincott Williams & Wilkins, 2009: 295–304.
Verebey KG and Meenan G, Diagnostic laboratory: screening for drug abuse. In *Lowinson and Ruiz's Substance Abuse: A Comprehensive Textbook*. Philadelphia: Wolters Kluwer, Lippincott Williams & Wilkins, 2011.

Alcohol is not usually part of urine drug testing because it is only detectable in the urine for a very short time—around 9 hours—depending on the quantity and chronicity of alcohol consumption. Blood or breath alcohol testing give a better idea of a person's alcohol level, but the window of detection is shorter.

With the various labs and collection methods, it can be difficult to decide which test to order for which patient. Here's my bottom-line advice:
• If you have no collection facility at your office, I suggest working with

one or more local lab collection sites. Large national laboratory service companies such as LabCorp or Quest Diagnostics have multiple collection sites in many areas and are usually set up to do urine collection for drug testing. Which lab(s) you send patients to will often depend on the individual patient's health insurance. Just fill out a lab order requisition (available online or through an electronic health record system) and give it to the patient or send it to the lab.

• If you have a collection facility, the on-site lab can often help you determine what tests to order.

Blood

Blood sampling is an accurate way of determining how much of a drug is in a patient's system, but its detection window is only 6–12 hours, so it's hard to use for random screens unless you can draw the sample in your office.

Hair

Hair analysis gives you a much wider detection window (up to 90 days) and is an easy and noninvasive collection method. However, it won't tell you about your patient's current substance use (it doesn't detect use within the previous 7–10 days), and it can't detect alcohol use. Other limitations of hair testing include difficulty in detecting low-level (single-time) use, and potential inaccuracy depending on your patient's hair color (some drugs have enhanced binding to melanin in dark hair). While it's hard to adulterate a hair sample, some patients may bleach their hair or shave their head to avoid this kind of testing; if so, hair on any other part of the body can be used.

Saliva

A quick swab of the inner cheek provides easy collection for saliva, which can be used to detect traces of drugs and alcohol. Oral fluid testing is comparable to urine testing and is less invasive; it's also harder for patients to adulterate or substitute. However, not all labs are equipped to test this type of sample.

Sweat

A skin patch that looks like a large adhesive bandage can be worn by patients for up to 7–14 days to measure drugs in their sweat. This has become a popular way for parole programs to monitor drug use. It's noninvasive, easily administered, and hard to adulterate (unless the patient removes the patch). This method is limited by the availability of testing facilities; it's also not entirely clear whether its results are affected by how much a person sweats. Commercial manufacturers have developed several wearable detection devices to monitor blood alcohol level; these are primarily aimed at consumers who are worried about getting a DUI, so they can plan to limit their alcohol consumption or find a ride home.

Nails

Drug testing from nails is rare compared to testing of urine, hair, or oral fluid. Similar to hair testing, nail testing has a long window of detection. However, not many labs test nails, and there is insufficient scientific data to support its routine use. Other limitations include the risk of environmental contamination of nails for some drug classes; nail testing also cannot detect alcohol.

Breath

Not every clinic needs an alcohol breathalyzer, but it can be helpful if you think your patient has been drinking and you need to consider safety issues (such as whether the patient should drive). The patient blows into a breathalyzer device, which returns a number representing the patient's blood alcohol concentration. A breathalyzer's detection window is similar to blood testing (6–12 hours), but varies depending on the amount of alcohol consumed over time. Some court systems mandate alcohol breathalyzer ignition interlocks for the vehicles of DUI offenders, which prevent the car from being started if the breath alcohol level is too high.

COLLECTING THE SAMPLE

Most office-based psychiatrists will send their patients to a lab for both urine collection and testing. But in case you decide to in-source some drug testing duties, here are some tips and best practices.

How some patients try to cheat urine tests

A cottage industry now caters to clients who want to game the system and hide their drug use from doctors and employers. There are a myriad of urine test cheating techniques, and new ones appear regularly. Here are a few of the more common methods:

- Waiting just long enough before giving a sample so that the drug is no longer detectable
- Switching one's urine with a sample from a clean donor ("clean pee" as it's known on the black market)
- Altering one's urine with additives such as aspirin, Drano, hydrogen peroxide, lemon juice, vinegar, liquid soap . . . the list goes on, and patients can look up sources and instructions on the internet
- Diluting urine with water
- Synthetic urine devices that might fool a monitor observing the production of a sample

> **FUN FACT: The Whizzinator**
>
> For about $140, patients can order the Whizzinator, a fake penis that comes with two leg straps and a waistband to "be sure everything stays in place," according to its website. The device features heating pads to ensure a realistic liquid temperature and includes a vial of the highest-quality synthetic urine. (http://www.thewhizzinator.com/)

Best practices for urine collection

You can outsmart aspiring cheaters by establishing good procedures for collecting urine. The Department of Transportation (DOT) has been helpful in developing some of these protocols, because it is the federal organization responsible for drug-testing people in potentially hazardous occupations, such as long-distance truck drivers. While there is no requirement that you follow DOT procedures, many clinics do, and it's helpful to understand their protocol as you create your own procedures.

Ideally, you should have a dedicated restroom for urine collection, one in which there is no access to tap or toilet water. This decreases the chance that a patient will dilute the urine sample. Patients should not be allowed to take anything with them into the restroom, like a coat, purse, or briefcase, and they should be asked to empty their pockets. This is to prevent smuggling in an adulterant or their own previously produced clean urine sample. Often a same-sex monitor will observe the sample being produced.

In my clinic, I initially give my patients the benefit of the doubt and let them produce the sample privately. However, if the staff doing the collecting has any concerns about the sample (for example, the patient took a really long time or was too quick, or the sample seemed too cool for normal body temperature), we will immediately request another sample, which *is* directly observed.

Preliminary testing

Before sending a sample to the lab, we usually do dipstick testing to ensure the patient has not tampered with the sample. A test strip is dipped in the urine and then compared to a color chart after 1 minute. We check for the following results:

- *pH.* Normal urine has a pH range of 4.5–8 (normal is around 6.0). If the pH is too low, the patient may have adulterated the sample. In one case, a patient provided a sample of very low pH, and it turned out to be pure lemonade. In addition to the low pH, as you can imagine, the glucose was off the charts! If the pH is too high (meaning too alkaline or basic), sometimes this means it was adulterated with bleach, which patients may do because the bleach interferes with the assay for cocaine, causing a false negative.
- *Specific gravity.* Specific gravity is a measure of urine concentration. The normal range is 1.0030–1.0300 (water is 1.000). The typical problem is that the specific gravity is too low, which happens when patients drink a lot of water prior to testing. The point of "water loading" is to dilute urine as much as possible so that the concentration of the substance will be below the lowest level of detection. If the specific gravity is so low that it is not consistent with human urine, this usually means the patient poured water directly into the collection cup—an argument for following the DOT protocol of providing a water-free restroom for collection. If the urine has high specific gravity, this usually means dehydration, more common in summer months.

The timing of testing

When I order testing, I ask patients to get it done that same day, but I will give them 48 hours if needed. Most drugs take more than 48 hours to be cleared from the urine. I typically say, "Here is your lab slip. You should go to the lab today to give a urine sample, although if that's not possible, you have up to 48 hours." When I receive the results, I'll compare the collection time listed on the lab sheet with the date and time of my note. If the testing occurred after more than 48 hours, I'll have a discussion with the patient at the next visit.

Lab analysis and confirmatory testing

Most labs will do an immunoassay for screening. During this process, antibodies to specific antigens are added to the urine sample. If any antibodies bind to drugs, these reactions are identified and reported. The downside of the immunoassay is that it only screens for a limited number of chemicals, depending on how many antibodies are used for different drugs. This can cause a false negative test. Conversely, some of the antibodies can cross-react with chemicals that are similar but not identical to the substance of interest, which would lead to a false positive.

When you want to be certain of what is in your patient's urine, you can order confirmatory testing (CT). The most common CT is gas chromatography/mass spectrometry. If CT reports the presence of a drug, there is no disputing that the drug was in the patient's system at some point. The downside is that these tests take longer and are more expensive; insurance companies will typically require patients to shoulder some of that expense. My practice is to do CT with the first sample in all my patients, and afterwards I will order it randomly. If the patient has had frequent positive urine screens, I will order CT more often. Since this can be a significant expense for patients, it offers a financial incentive for them to avoid relapsing.

Easy point-of-care testing

The easiest way to do point-of-care (POC) testing in your office is with all-in-one commercially available kits that provide results in less than 5 minutes, similar to a urine pregnancy test. The urine collection cups often have the reagents inside the cup wall or lid so that you don't have to dip in a strip and expose office staff to the urine—you just look at the markings that appear on the closed cup to read the results. The downside is that you can only test for the drugs that the kits are equipped to detect.

TEST RESULTS

CASE REVISITED: *D returns for a follow-up appointment 2 weeks later. You open his chart and see the results of his urine drug screen: He tested positive for both THC and amphetamines. You are dismayed, because you feel that*

he was not forthcoming with you during your initial interview. But you're
not sure how to discuss the results of the test without sounding like a cop.

False positives

Before you discuss lab results with your patient, you should understand
the limitations of the testing process, such as false positives. Actual false
positives are quite rare—if you get a positive drug test, the likelihood is
extremely high that your patient is using that substance. That said, there are
a small number of potential positive screens that are caused by legitimate
use of prescribed or over-the-counter (OTC) drugs (see Table 2-3). The
package insert that comes with a manufacturer's immunoassay will list the
compounds most likely to cause a false positive. If there is any doubt, call the
manufacturer's customer service, or talk with the lab that performed the test.

Opioids

Ask whether the patient has been taking Tylenol #3, which patients
may not realize is Tylenol with codeine. Fluoroquinolones are a class of
commonly prescribed antibiotics that include levofloxacin (Levaquin),

TABLE 2-3. False Positives on Drug Screens

Drug	Potential Cause of False Positive	Notes
Opioids	• Tylenol #3 with codeine • Poppy seeds • Fluoroquinolones (levofloxacin, ofloxacin, gatifloxacin)	May be legitimate prescription
Amphetamine	• Adderall (levo-amphetamine and dextro-amphetamine) • Vyvanse (lisdexamphetamine) • Eldepryl (selegiline) • Vicks VapoInhaler	May be legitimate prescription Prescribed for Parkinson's disease; metabolizes to levo-amphetamine OTC, contains levo-methamphetamine
Barbiturates	• Fiorinal/Fioricet (butalbital) • Donnatal (phenobarbital)	May be legitimate prescriptions
Cocaine	TAC solution (tetracaine, adrenaline, and cocaine)	Used as local anesthetic for suturing lacerations
THC	Marinol (dronabinol)	May be legitimate prescription
Phencyclidine	• Dextromethorphan • Effexor (venlafaxine)	May cross-react with immunoassay

ofloxacin (Floxin), and gatifloxacin (Tequin); they may cross-react with an immunoassay for opioids, but this is not always true for every commercially available immunoassay.

Benzodiazepines

Not all benzodiazepines are detected on drug screens. Alprazolam and diazepam, the most commonly misused benzodiazepines, are reliably detected. Lorazepam and chlordiazepoxide are sporadically detected, and clonazepam is often not picked up. Sometimes when I see unexpected positive results for benzodiazepines, the patients are legitimately receiving the medications from another doctor and do not realize they are potentially abusable. I make sure they recognize the issue, and this usually offers a teaching opportunity about the disadvantages of taking a benzodiazepine while struggling with recovery from another drug.

Stimulants

Some OTC preparations can cause false positives for stimulants, such as pseudoephedrine, but a patient will have had to ingest several boxes of it to produce a false positive. Vicks VapoInhaler is an OTC product in a plastic lipstick-size tube that contains levo-methamphetamine (a racemic isomer of methamphetamine that is not psychoactive), which can cause a false positive result for amphetamines. The cocaine assay is very reliable—there are very few false positives, and it doesn't cross-react with lidocaine or Novocaine.

Phencyclidine

Phencyclidine (PCP) false positives are possible from dextromethorphan in OTC cough medications, and from some antipsychotics.

False negatives

False negatives are more common than false positives, since patients who are continuing to use despite treatment have a strong incentive to be creative in efforts to mask their use—and there is a robust internet-based industry catering to this market (see Table 2-4).

The most common way of achieving a false negative is water loading, which I discussed earlier. There are various other readily available substances that can be used to adulterate a urine sample. For example, patients can add table salt to a sample, which can be effective, but if they add too

TABLE 2-4. False Negatives on Drug Screens

Potential Cause of False Negative	Drugs Masked	Notes
Visine OTC eye drops (tetrahydrozoline)	THC benzodiazepines	Visine is squirted into urine cup (squirting in eyes is not effective for urine)
Drano or laundry bleach (sodium hypochlorite)	amphetamine barbiturates benzodiazepines cocaine opiates THC	Increases pH, but may cause visible foam in urine
Vinegar (acetic acid)	THC	Lowers pH of urine sample
Ammonia	multiple, depends on assay	Increases pH, has characteristic smell
Table salt (sodium chloride)	amphetamine barbiturate cocaine opiates THC	Increases specific gravity of urine sample (>1.035), may precipitate out
Hydrogen peroxide	THC opiates LSD	May cause bubbles in urine
Liquid hand soap	multiple, depends on assay	May cause bubbles or make urine cloudy
Glutaraldehyde (UrinAid)	cocaine amphetamine barbiturates benzodiazepines opiates THC	Internet purchase, some labs may test for this adulterant
Pyridinium chlorochromate (Urine Luck)	opiates THC	Internet purchase
Potassium nitrite (Klear, Whizzies)	THC	Internet purchase

much it can precipitate out and make the effort obvious. Vinegar will mask THC testing, but it lowers the pH of the urine sample, which will be picked up on dipstick testing or by the lab in more formal testing. Other specialized adulterants are available on the internet, usually selling for about $19.99 per use. Some labs will test for the more common adulterants like glutaraldehyde. The marketing for these products can be amusing. For example, the product "Urine Luck" hired Tommy Chong (from Cheech and Chong) to deliver the memorable slogan, "When you're caught with your pants down, Urine Luck."

Discussing problematic results

Depending on your expectations, you may or may not be surprised when you receive positive results from a patient's drug screening. It can be challenging to share this initial news. Sometimes I frame it as a question so the patients feel comfortable sharing the information with me. For example, if a patient's urine is positive, I might say, "Your urine had a positive result; can you tell me about that?" Sometimes, instead of the word "positive," I'll say "concerning" or "problematic." Other times I'll just come straight out and tell the patient what was found: "Your most recent urine drug test was positive for pot and cocaine. Can you help me understand that?"

> ### ⬤ CLINICAL PEARL: Don't Call It "Dirty"
> *People often use the terms "clean urine" or "dirty urine," but there's a move to get away from these types of stigmatizing terms. I tend to use terms like "problematic," "positive," or "expected vs. unexpected" results. You wouldn't say a "dirty urine" came back if a urine test for a diabetic patient revealed high amounts of sugar—you'd tell the patient that the disease is not under good control, and you'd make the appropriate therapeutic decisions. It's helpful to adopt a similar mindset when talking to patients about urine drug test results.*

In the best-case scenario, your patient will respond by admitting the use of the drug; if so, this presents a great opportunity to explore what caused the use. Ask where it occurred, whether there was a craving, and whether there was a specific trigger.

CASE REVISITED: *You look up from the urine drug screen results and say to D, "I got your drug screen report back, and it looks like there were a couple of positive results."*

D responds, "Is it the pot? I don't know if I told you about using pot sometimes; I actually have a medical use card that I got a few months ago for headaches and anxiety."

"I see. Yes, there was THC, and there was also amphetamine."

"Amphetamine?" asks D. "You mean like snorting meth? I don't do that."

"It could come from a medication like Ritalin or Adderall."

"Oh, okay—it must be Adderall, then. Sometimes I use my wife's Adderall for depression."

This leads to a productive discussion about alternatives to Adderall and marijuana for dealing with D's depressed moods.

Disputing test results

Sometimes, patients dispute positive tests. Here are a couple of common patient responses to positive drug screens, along with suggestions for how you might deal with these situations most effectively.

1. Patient disputes validity of result

"I don't know how that got there."
"That can't be right."
"Somebody must have switched urines on me."
"The lab must have mixed up the samples."

Clinician Response: Generally I give the patient the benefit of the doubt rather than arguing about the specific result. But if it happens more than once, I will discuss my concern with the patient. I might say, "While there are documented cases of labs handling samples improperly, these are quite rare— professional labs have rigorous systems in place to prevent errors. If you are disputing this, though, we can have you give another sample right away."

2. Patient claims the substance entered the bloodstream but didn't actually "use" it

"I was in a room where people were smoking pot, but I didn't use it myself."
"I was just handling the drug, but I didn't use it."
"I had sex with a guy who had just used it."

Clinician Response: The science is clear that false positives without using are extremely unlikely. For example, one study estimated that for there to be a false positive due to secondhand smoke, a person would have had to be sitting next to smokers in a poorly ventilated small car driving for two days across the country. The other issue is that labs have high detection thresholds, which means that for a substance to be detectable, a person's urine would need to contain so much of the substance that the person would have noticed a clinical effect—in other words, the person would have been high. However, I don't go into these debates with patients because I don't want the visit to be adversarial. Instead, I will say something like, "Well, if you're working on your recovery, it's probably not good for you to put yourself in a situation where others around you are using."

Once a patient who tested positive for cocaine said, "Someone must have sprinkled some cocaine in my drink." My response was, "Be careful of your friends, and keep an eye on your drink!"

> ### FUN FACT: MROs: The Ultimate Experts on Drug Testing
> In this chapter, I've only exposed you to the tip of the drug-testing iceberg. Interpreting tests can become quite complicated, and physicians interested in the subject can become certified as a medical review officer (MRO). The training takes two to three days and culminates in an exam. MROs work with various organizations that do employee drug testing, such as businesses and federal agencies. I received my MRO certification in 1999. One of the ways we help is serving as intermediaries between an employee and a business. If an employee has a positive result, that result will go directly and confidentially to an MRO before going to the employer. This enables the MRO to ask the employee about the result, and if the employee can explain it, the MRO will report a negative test to the employer.

How often should you order drug tests?

How often to order drug screens is a judgment call that will depend on your practice and patient mix. One reason for doing more frequent testing initially is that patients are less likely to be stable early in treatment, and frequent testing allows for quicker detection of problems. But another reason relates to the credit analogy—patients with frequent, negative test results early on have a chance to quickly build up "good credit."

For a typical patient, I will usually order testing at each appointment for the first two or three visits, then at every other appointment for the next three to four months. If the patient remains stable, I will further spread out the testing intervals to monthly, quarterly, or more. Although clinicians have their own time tables, there is a federal standard for federally funded methadone clinics, where stable patients are mandated to receive drug testing a minimum of 8 times per year.

How should you announce to a patient that today will be a drug test day? Generally, I mention it close to the end of the visit, saying something like, "We're going to get a urine tox screen today; is there anything that you forgot to tell me?" I've found that if you announce the test at the beginning of the appointment, patients tend to get nervous, which might mean they are worried about the result.

CASE CONCLUSION: *D agrees that his Adderall use is likely worsening his bipolar mood shifts and says he will try to discontinue his occasional use. He agrees to getting urine drug screens on a random basis in the future.*

Self-Test Questions

1. You recently started seeing a patient for generalized anxiety disorder, and you are continuing his clonazepam 0.5 mg twice daily, which was started by a previous psychiatrist. You order a urine drug screen, and the result comes back negative for benzodiazepines. Which of the following is the most likely explanation for this result?
   a. The patient's dose of clonazepam is below the drug screen's detection level
   b. Not all benzodiazepines are detected on a urine drug screen immuno-assay
   c. The patient diluted his urine sample
   d. The patient adulterated his urine sample with potassium nitrite

2. A 45-year-old woman is being monitored for alcohol use disorder through an employee assistance program. Her most recent urine drug immunoassay was positive for opiates. The patient denies taking any opiates, but states that she started taking a new medication just before her last urine drug screen. Which of the following medications is the most likely cause of this false positive?
   a. Imipramine
   b. Ketorolac

   c. Ofloxacin

   d. Selegiline

3. Which of the following substances, when used once, will be detectable for the longest time in a urine sample?

   a. Alcohol

   b. Lorazepam

   c. Marijuana

   d. Phencyclidine

The answer key for these self-test questions is on page 233.

Note: If you purchased CME credit with this book, your CME post-test can be accessed when you are logged in at www.thecarlatreport.com/AddictionGuide. Please keep in mind that the question and answer order for that CME post-test are different than what you see in these self-test study questions.

CHAPTER 3

Understanding Addiction Services

"I guess the worst day I have had was when I had to
stand up in rehab in front of my wife and daughter
and say, 'Hi, my name is Sam, and I am an addict.' "
Samuel L. Jackson, actor

(Some of the material in this chapter was adapted from an article written by Susan Hochstedler for the *Carlat Addiction Treatment Report*, August 2015.)

TAKE HOME POINTS

- Outpatient treatment with an addiction specialist is sufficient for many patients.
- A 3- to 7-day inpatient detox is often the gateway for more intensive treatment.
- Intensive outpatient programs are 3 sessions per week and good for those who have a job.
- Partial hospitalization programs are 5 full days per week and include daily meetings with a psychopharmacologist.
- Residential rehabs are 30-day programs that are often expensive and for people who cannot maintain sobriety anywhere else.

CASE VIGNETTE: *Your patient, M, is a 28-year-old woman with panic disorder whom you have treated for 3 years. She had called you for an urgent appointment, and today she informs you that she was released 4 days ago from a detox facility where she was admitted for opioid use disorder. After registering your surprise (she had never told you about her opioid addiction, saying she was embarrassed about it), you establish that she had been addicted to OxyContin for 6 months, and that she had entered detox at the urging of her parents. M states she has not had any opioids* *since discharge, but that she has severe cravings to use. At the hospital, she was approached by a representative of a large company that operates residential rehab facilities, and the rep urged her parents to admit her to one. However, M's health insurance is not accepted by these programs, and the out-of-pocket payment is $50,000–$60,000 per month, depending on the facility. Your patient's family is well off, but they are reluctant to pay this amount of money. M is asking you for advice. Should her family bite the bullet and fund a residential facility, or are there other options? M makes it clear she wants treatment, but would prefer not to be admitted to another facility, since she had a somewhat difficult experience in the detox unit.*

INTRODUCTION

For a variety of economic and historical reasons, the U.S. substance use treatment system has become quite complicated, and in some cases separated from the rest of psychiatry. This means that the general clinician may not understand the treatment options available. To make matters worse, a strong profit motive has led to the mushrooming of expensive residential rehab centers, which can run well above the $50,000-per-month figure quoted to your patient, M.

In some cases, you won't be particularly involved in deciding what treatment a patient receives; such choices are often made in the setting of a substance use treatment program, usually during or after an acute detox. Nonetheless, it's helpful for you to have an overview of treatment options available for substance-using patients. In some cases, your patient will ask you for advice, and in others, you will be contacted by a treatment setting about your patient; for both scenarios, you will want a clear idea of where a program fits in the context of treatment settings.

SPECIALIST CLINICIANS

Before describing the programs, let's go over the variety of health care professionals specializing in substance use treatment. You are likely to have contact with many of them during your career.

Addiction counselors and therapists

There are many therapists with an interest or certification in addictions. The most well-known national certifying organization is NAADAC, The

USEFUL FACT: The ASAM Criteria

The ASAM criteria are the American Society of Addiction Medicine's guidelines for matching severity of illness and level of function with intensity of service in addiction treatment. Treatment matching means providing the patient with the least restrictive level of care that is likely to be beneficial. This involves assessing people in six dimensions and matching them with the most appropriate level of care so that services are provided in the most efficient manner. Criteria such as these help clinicians determine and justify whether a patient requires outpatient or residential or inpatient services with medical monitoring (for treatment of withdrawal or comorbidities).

The ASAM criteria are used primarily by addiction specialists who need to demonstrate to insurance companies that a certain level of care is needed. For more details on incorporating the ASAM criteria into your practice, see the *Carlat Addiction Treatment Report*, November 2014.

Association for Addiction Professionals (formerly called the National Association for Alcoholism and Drug Abuse Counselors). The training requirements for such certified counselors vary from state to state. For example, in Texas, where I work, such counselors are called licensed chemical dependency counselors, and their training entails having at least an associate degree, completing 4,000 hours of supervised experience treating patients with substance use disorders, then passing a state certification examination to obtain a state license. You will typically find these counselors working in rehab programs or intensive outpatient programs.

Going up the ladder of training requirements, there are clinical social workers (who generally have a master's degree in social work) and clinical psychologists (who have a PhD or PsyD). Some therapists specialize exclusively in addiction treatment, some have general practices that include addiction treatment, and others will not treat addiction specifically but will address issues related to relationships, coping skills, etc, all of which might be useful for your patients. I recommend that you develop a list of good local practitioners to whom you can refer patients. You can assemble this list based on feedback from your patients or from colleagues.

Specialist physicians

You will likely need to refer some patients to physicians who specialize in addiction. There are two addiction specialties for MDs: addiction medicine, open to all specialties, and addiction psychiatry, open only to psychiatrists. An addiction psychiatry specialist completes a one-year fellowship in addiction psychiatry after residency, and then passes a certification exam conducted by the American Academy of Addiction Psychiatry. An addiction medicine specialist must complete a residency in any medical specialty (psychiatry, internal medicine, family medicine, pediatrics, preventive medicine, obstetrics, etc) and then complete a fellowship in addiction medicine, or demonstrate substantial time spent delivering substance abuse care (after 2022, only those who have completed a fellowship in addiction medicine will be eligible for certification).

Interventionists

Interventionists are addiction professionals who specialize in orchestrating the sometimes-dramatic interventions that have become fodder for reality TV shows. Usually it is the emotionally exhausted family that seeks this kind of help. An interventionist generally offers three services: planning and executing the intervention, finding an appropriate treatment program for the patient, and providing "recovery coaching" after treatment, often for a year or more. There's usually a fee for each service, and insurance rarely if ever pays for it. (You can get some good insight into what it's like to work as an interventionist in the August 2015 issue of the *Carlat Addiction Treatment Report*, which includes an interview with Paul Gallant, an intervention professional.)

 DID YOU KNOW? How to Find an Addiction Specialist

A great resource for locating addiction specialists in your area is the SAMHSA treatment locator (https://findtreatment.samhsa.gov). Just type in your ZIP code, and you'll get a list of nearby facilities.

To find a prescriber for buprenorphine, use the Buprenorphine Treatment Physician Locator (buprenorphine.samhsa.gov), which is searchable by state, city, or ZIP code.

GROUP/INSTITUTIONAL/HOSPITAL PROGRAMS

12-step programs

We devote a chapter to the topic of 12-step programs, but as an introduction you should know that these are nonprofessional mutual self-help groups that are community-organized and free. They aren't considered treatments per se because they don't involve licensed counselors providing care to patients. Nonetheless, 12-step programs are often the first form of help that substance-using patients seek out. Many clinicians will view a referral to AA meetings as a convenient first step.

The following section details the types of addiction treatment services available (see Table 3-1).

Detox

Detox is the process of quickly getting a patient off drugs or alcohol. It's often a prelude to rehab since it's hard for patients to make headway in recovery while they are actively using. While detox can be either outpatient or inpatient, inpatient treatment is the best choice for those withdrawing

TABLE 3-1. Available Addiction Treatment Services

Format	Description	Duration	Staffing/Programming
Detox	Get patients off substances	5–7 days for alcohol, 3–5 days for opioids	Hospital setting with counselors, nurses, physicians
Intensive outpatient treatment	Outpatient treatment that can accommodate job and family obligations	4–8 weeks total, often 9 hours per week, spread out over 3 days	Office setting with substance abuse counselors
Partial hospitalization program	"Full-time" outpatient treatment	2–3 weeks, 5 days per week, 6 hours per day	Hospital setting with counselors, nurses, psychopharmacologists
Residential rehab	For those with toxic home environments and who have consistently failed outpatient treatment	30 days, residential	Group and individual treatments with professional counselors and other activities; most include 12-step meetings on site
Long-term residential (aka therapeutic communities and recovery houses)	For patients who relapse frequently and need long-term structure	6–12 months, residential	Similar staffing and programming as 30-day rehab with more emphasis on peer counselors in good recovery
Sober houses (aka halfway houses)	Independent living arrangement with minimal staffing	1–2 years, residential	Residents expected to attend many community 12-step meetings; weekly urine drug testing
Holding beds (aka transitional stabilization units)	Bare-bones residential facility while waiting for rehab placement	Up to several months	Minimal programming; some counseling and 12-step meetings

from substantial daily alcohol use (such as a pint of hard liquor or 12–24 beers per day), and for those with concurrent or preexisting medical problems, such as heart or liver disease. How do you get patients into detox? If you know some detox facilities in your area, the best route is to call them directly (or have the patient or family call). Some centers will do their own screening, whereas others will require the patient to visit the ER before referral. Obviously, most patients will prefer to bypass the ER. Another option is to start by calling the insurance company: It will provide the names of local detox programs with which it contracts, and the company may have specific hoops to jump through before it will authorize treatment.

> **CLINICAL PEARL: How Long Does Inpatient Detox Last?**
> *If you refer patients to detox, they will often want to know how long it will last. While each patient's experience will vary, inpatient detox usually lasts 5–7 days for both alcohol and benzodiazepines and 3–5 days for opioids.*

Intensive outpatient programs (IOP)

IOP usually consists of 9 hours per week of outpatient treatment, divided into three 3-hour sessions. They are generally group therapy sessions that offer rehabilitative counseling and educational classes. These programs are offered in either day or evening formats. IOP is a good option for people who are struggling with sobriety after detox, or for those whose job or family obligations prevent more time-intensive treatment. In some cases, the person's insurance may only cover IOP.

In contrast to 12-step programs, IOPs are professionally facilitated groups, and they can be uniquely helpful for patients on several levels. Whereas in a one-on-one setting, patients might feel uncomfortable talking about certain behaviors, a group offers a sense of mutual permission and support. And unlike self-help groups such as AA, having a facilitator in charge can keep people on task and prevent certain individuals from monopolizing the conversation.

Partial hospitalization programs (PHP)

Also known as "day treatment," PHPs usually run 5 days a week, 6 hours per day, and last 10–15 days. These programs are much more comprehensive than IOPs. They tend to have more sophisticated therapy groups, such as dialectical behavior therapy, cognitive behavioral therapy, and family therapy. Psychopharmacologists are also on staff for appointments as part of the daily treatment program. Insurance companies will approve PHP primarily for patients with comorbid psychiatric disorders.

Residential rehab

Residential rehabilitation programs are 30-day inpatient programs that vary widely in cost, philosophy, and personnel. Residential rehab is for patients who have a toxic or unsupportive home environment—they may live alone or have family members who are actively using. Residential rehab is also appropriate for people who have repeatedly relapsed at a lower level of care. The classic rehab is a pricey, for-profit company providing a luxurious environment and requiring payment up front; such programs can run $50,000 per month or more. Less pricey than residential rehab are 12-step immersion programs, which clock in at around $10,000 per month. These facilities can actually be fairly luxurious (think big lodges and beautiful farms); they are cheaper because they are run primarily by people in recovery and by addiction counselors without advanced degrees. The programming in 12-step immersion is limited to AA—from the moment patients walk in, they will be doing AA steps. Finally, there are some bare-bones residential rehabs covered by Medicaid. For some patients, being in a less ritzy setting can serve as a motivator to avoid future rehab stints.

FUN FACT: The Word's Ritziest Rehab

The world's most expensive residential rehab program is not located in Malibu, but on the shores of Lake Zurich, in Switzerland. Kusnacht Practice costs $100,000 per week. The facility treats one patient at a time, greets clients at the airport with a personal driver, and provides butlers, personal chefs, personal trainers, and yoga teachers. Twelve specialists devise a treatment plan for each well-heeled patient, and their focus is on "biomolecular restoration," a process that includes "comprehensive laboratory testing" leading to a "personalized organic formulation, comprising micronutrients and amino acids," according to the practice's website (http://kusnachtpractice.com).

CASE REVISITED: *M's parents are letting her stay at their house while she receives substance use treatment. She has a job as a waitress that she does not want to lose. Given that M appears motivated and has a supportive home environment, you tell her that she does not need a residential rehab facility. You recommend either a PHP or an IOP. M and her family choose the IOP, and you strongly recommend that she also attend NA (Narcotics Anonymous) meetings and meet with a psychopharmacologist affiliated with the IOP who can evaluate her for possible medication-assisted treatment with buprenorphine.*

Long-term residential

These programs are also known as therapeutic communities or recovery house. They last 6–12 months, and are for people who relapse so frequently that they need to be away from their community and spend significant time in a very structured environment. They learn to incorporate recovery skills in their lives and gain the self-esteem and confidence to create a network of people they can depend on when they're stressed. Some long-term residential programs are called "working houses" because they have a return-to-work requirement after 1 to 2 months.

Sober houses

A sober house, also called a halfway house, is an independent living arrangement with minor oversight where residents can stay for 1–2 years. Most of these residencies have a house manager, but they lack on-site professional counselors or programming. Residents are sometimes told, "Here's your key; you can come and go as you want, but everyone here is sober." At some houses, there is a curfew or restrictions on weekends away, especially for newcomers. At others, individuals may move up along a "levels" system, gaining more privileges with each level. Residents are expected to attend outside 12-step meetings frequently, at least 4 times a week, and to undergo weekly random drug testing. As part of the living arrangement, some sober houses require that residents find at least part-time work in the community. Sober houses are often a good segue from a residential program, because they provide support within the community environment and teach people to take more responsibility for their recovery. Some people find that they cannot maintain sobriety outside of sober houses.

Holding beds

Sadly, there is a countrywide shortage of residential beds. Because of this, there are many transitional stabilization units, otherwise known as holding beds. They are usually federally funded, and they provide a bare-bones facility for people to stay while they wait for residential beds. The usual occupant of a holding bed is a recently detoxed patient who needs residential treatment to maintain sobriety, but does not have the necessary funds for a rehab program, even one of the cheaper options. People may stay here for up to a few months as they wait for a placement.

Court-mandated treatment

Referring patients to treatment is all well and good, but up to a third of patients in rehab facilities are there by court order, usually involuntarily. As a clinician, you might be involved in the process of forcing a patient into treatment, so it's important to understand the process.

Many states (but not all) have a provision allowing court-mandated treatment. In Massachusetts, the process is called a "section 35," which refers to a section of the state law. This provision is used for patients who are out of control with their use but refuse treatment. Most of the time in this scenario, you have the family coming to you asking, "What can we do, Doctor?" They explain the ways in which their family member is engaging in risky behavior or endangering others, such as, "He's falling and hurting himself when he's drunk" or, "She overdosed on heroin and we barely got her to the ER on time." At this point, you need to intervene to keep the person safe.

The procedure is as follows. The family has to prepare a case for involuntary commitment. It will be in the form of testimony, but it is often augmented by medical reports and even photographic evidence (I advise these families to keep their phones at the ready and take video of the intoxicated behavior). A hearing is scheduled at which a judge weighs the evidence; if the judge agrees that the situation is dire, a writ of apprehension will be issued. The police will then bring the person in handcuffs to court, where the patient hears the evidence, has a chance to refute it before the judge, and expresses willingness (or unwillingness) to enter treatment. If committed involuntarily, the person will be taken to a state-funded residential rehab facility for up to 90 days. Do such involuntary commitments work? Often not so much. Patients can be released early if they agree to outpatient counseling and AA meetings, but this may be a ruse for getting back to substance use. Nonetheless, involuntary commitment does give the family some respite, and it creates the chance, no matter how small, that the patient will eventually buy into the need for treatment.

Court-mandated treatment can be initiated by the family, the police, or any physician. The limiting factor is the requirement to go to court—something physicians are rarely willing to do. You might be surprised to learn, however, that involuntary commitment has similar outcomes to voluntary treatment when looking at long-term success rates. Patients can still learn from and benefit from treatment, even if they grumble about having to be there.

A final word of advice—I recommend getting to know the treatment centers and providers in your area. Go to a local IOP or PHP and sit in on a staff meeting. The more working relationships you have with addiction professionals, the more efficient you will be at referring your patient to the right treatment, at the right place, and at the right time.

CASE CONCLUSION: *A week after your appointment with M, you get a call from her parents. M did follow up with an IOP, but at her waitressing job, she ran into a friend who offered her some Vicodin after work, and she relapsed. The IOP's director referred her to a local PHP, where she will attend programs daily and be seen by a psychopharmacologist for buprenorphine treatment. You will begin treating M again in about a month, after she finishes her PHP.*

Self-Test Questions

1. Compared with a patient who voluntarily enters an addiction treatment program, how likely is a patient who enters court-mandated treatment to experience a sustained period of recovery?
   a. More likely
   b. Less likely
   c. Equally as likely
   d. Not enough data available

2. A 53-year-old man enters a treatment program for his alcohol use disorder. In this type of program, participants are expected to work with peer counselors and staff members who demonstrate appropriate recovery

behaviors and act as role models. The patient is initially assigned to menial jobs, but after 2 years, he has progressed in recovery and worked his way up to tasks with authority, finally becoming a staff member himself. This type of substance use treatment program is known as which of the following?

a. Intensive outpatient program

b. Motivational enhancement therapy

c. Mutual self-help group

d. Therapeutic community

3. Which of the following therapists completes the most professional training prior to obtaining licensure?

a. Licensed chemical dependency counselor

b. Peer counselor

c. Clinical psychologist

d. Social worker

The answer key for these self-test questions is on page 233.

Note: If you purchased CME credit with this book, your CME post-test can be accessed when you are logged in at www.thecarlatreport.com/AddictionGuide. Please keep in mind that the question and answer order for that CME post-test are different than what you see in these self-test study questions.

CHAPTER 4

Psychotherapy

"A lot of people think that addiction is a choice.
A lot of people think it's a matter of will. That
has not been my experience. I don't find it to
have anything to do with strength."
Matthew Perry, actor

TAKE HOME POINTS

- Use motivational interviewing to encourage self-motivational statements.
- Understand the five Stages of Change to recognize where your patient is on the spectrum of readiness to embrace recovery.
- Master the "good things and less-good things" and "typical day" techniques.
- Recognize when your patient is at risk for relapse and teach relapse prevention techniques, including refusal skills.
- Encourage your patient to journal daily and to share entries in sessions.

CASE VIGNETTE: *C is a 32-year-old female who started using cannabis in her early teens, first at parties with friends, then more regularly at home because it helped her relax when she felt anxious. About 2 years later, she tried cocaine and found that she liked it. She began using cocaine every weekend, then several times per week. Her retail job didn't leave her much money to spend on cocaine, but she had friends who were willing to give it to her most of the time. C continued to smoke cannabis, especially to help her feel better when she crashed after using cocaine. However, her anxiety was getting worse and was starting to affect her job performance. She contacted me for help with her use of cocaine and cannabis. In today's* *appointment, after discussing her drug use and anxiety symptoms, C expresses ambivalence about stopping these drugs entirely—especially cannabis, which she does not see as a problem.*

There are many types of therapy that are helpful for substance abusers. The most commonly used are cognitive behavioral therapy (CBT) and motivational interviewing; dialectical behavioral therapy is also gaining popularity. There is also relapse prevention therapy, which is an adaptation of CBT techniques specifically for substance abuse.

As a psychiatrist, you are unlikely to have the time to do traditional CBT, which includes specific techniques and usually is conducted in weekly or semiweekly 50-minute sessions. In this chapter, my focus will be on specific therapeutic techniques and skills that you can use in the context of your briefer 20- to 30-minute visits. This may entail a sort of grab bag of different techniques—it certainly has for my practice.

MOTIVATIONAL INTERVIEWING

Motivational interviewing (MI) was first developed for treating alcohol users, but it has since proven helpful for patients with a variety of psychiatric disorders. Its purpose is to help patients become aware of their intrinsic motivation to change their problematic behaviors. I find MI invaluable in helping my patients to accept substance use treatments such as detox or medication-assisted maintenance of sobriety/abstinence.

Stages of Change

The MI technique entails spending quite a bit of time assessing how ready your patient is to make significant changes. The Stages of Change model is a helpful theoretical framework to keep in mind while talking to patients, and I draw on it daily (see Table 4-1). According to the model, there are five stages of change: pre-contemplation, contemplation, preparation, action, and maintenance.

1. *Pre-contemplation.* This stage describes patients who don't yet see that there is any problem. Our job is to provide them with feedback based on what they are telling us about their lives. This often involves a summary statement such as, "It sounds like you've had these consequences related to your physical health, emotional health, finances, etc."

TABLE 4-1. Stages of Change

Pre-contemplation	Unaware that there is a problem
Contemplation	Aware of a problem, but not ready to change; will ask for information
Preparation	Considering a behavior change in the near future; will ask for advice
Action	Making a behavior change
Maintenance	Successfully changed behavior; using less energy to maintain the gains that have been made

As an example, I saw a 13-year-old girl who was brought in by her father because he was concerned about her alcohol and marijuana use. She did not want to be there, and said she didn't think she had a problem with substances. So I used some open-ended questions to learn a bit about her life, and then proceeded to more specific ones:

Doctor: What do you think your father is concerned about?

Patient: He thinks I shouldn't smoke any pot.

Doctor: Do you share his concerns?

Patient: I know that smoking pot can get me in trouble, but I don't think it's that bad.

I recognized this last assertion as a "self-motivational statement," meaning she volunteered that there was a negative consequence of her pot use. To feed back some of her concerns, I responded, "So you recognize that smoking pot may get you in trouble with your dad, but you don't see it as something that's really harmful to you otherwise."

Through the back-and-forth of our conversation, I learned that this patient was having depressive symptoms, such as anhedonia and irritability. She was clearly concerned about her depression, and she recognized that the drugs were not significantly improving her mood, though they made her feel better temporarily. She began to understand that continued use of drugs was likely to worsen her depressive symptoms, and I helped her to realize there were better alternatives. At the end of that first visit, she acknowledged that she might consider making some changes in her life. Using MI, I helped her move from the pre-contemplation to the contemplation stage.

2. *Contemplation.* In the contemplation stage, patients recognize that there's a problem, but they're not sure what to do. At this stage, they will typically ask for information to help them make a decision. Questions asked by patients in this stage include: "Doc, what does this mean for me?" "What if I keep on drinking—what could happen?" "Are there consequences that I may not be aware of?"

   You will often see a patient going through the contemplation stage in consultation-liaison psychiatry. For example, say a patient crashes his car because of drinking and is now in the hospital with some traumatic injuries. As a result of being powerfully confronted with the fact that his drinking has created a problem, he starts to contemplate whether he needs to get some treatment.

3. *Preparation.* In this stage, patients understand that there is a problem. They are beyond contemplation, and are ready to begin preparing to change. Preparation means patients are readying to make an abstinence attempt, but they haven't done much yet.

   For example, I saw a young woman in her early 20s who was spending too much money on drugs, had lost multiple jobs because of her addiction, and was living with her parents. She was worried about her health because she'd been injecting heroin, and her parents were not going to allow her to live with them unless she did something about her habit. At this point her chief complaint to me was, "I've gotten into trouble using heroin, especially mixed with fentanyl. I know I need to stop, but I don't know how to do it." She had moved beyond both contemplation and pre-contemplation, and was asking me for help as she prepared to take action. My strategy in such cases is to give patients a menu of options, rather than telling them what to do. This empowers them to make their own choice.

   In the case of this young woman, my assessment revealed that she wasn't using daily, but she was having some withdrawal symptoms. She was already on an antidepressant, and was using gabapentin (Neurontin) for anxiety. So I laid out three reasonable options for her. First, she could get onto buprenorphine with a plan to taper off of it; second, she could taper herself off the heroin at home, using gabapentin to help her do so; and third, she could go into a formal detox program. She elected to go with the second option, staying at home and using her prescribed

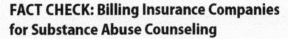

FACT CHECK: Billing Insurance Companies for Substance Abuse Counseling

Most psychiatrists are familiar with the basic CPT codes for psychotherapy, and for 20- to 30-minute visits, a common approach is to bill one of the E/M codes (99212, 99213, or 99214) and to add on a short psychotherapy code (90833). But you may not realize that there are also specific add-on codes for substance abuse and tobacco cessation counseling. Use these codes in addition to your usual office visit billing codes when you do screening (including with instruments discussed in Chapter 1 and in the Appendix) and/or brief intervention with a patient. Insurance companies and Medicaid/Medicare limit how often these add-on codes can be billed—usually 1–3 times per year.

Alcohol/substance use screening/intervention, 15–30 minutes – 99408

Alcohol/substance use screening/intervention, > 30 minutes – 99409

Alcohol/substance (other than tobacco) structured assessment (AUDIT, DAST) and brief intervention, 15–30 minutes – G0396

Alcohol/substance (other than tobacco) structured assessment (AUDIT, DAST) and brief intervention, > 30 minutes – G0397

Annual alcohol misuse screening, 15 minutes – G0442

Brief face-to-face behavioral counseling for alcohol misuse, 15 minutes – G0443

psychiatric meds to get over withdrawal. The patient felt that this was doable because it had been a couple of days since her last use, and she had not been using daily for several weeks. She declined the buprenorphine option because she had once had a rapid buprenorphine detox in a previous program that was unpleasant, and she didn't want to repeat that.

The patient's plan worked surprisingly well. Her symptoms subsided. She followed up a week later and told me she had met with a psychologist to discuss coping skills.

4. *Action.* People in the action stage are primed and ready. They have made a decision to get treatment, and you simply have to develop a treatment

plan for them to implement. I will discuss specifics of treatment plans in the chapters on substances later in this book.

5. *Maintenance.* In this stage, patients have made the initial quit attempt, and are now maintaining their recovery. For example, a patient may have completed an alcohol detox program, and attended 90 meetings in 90 days. Now he is in the maintenance phase of abstaining from drinking, going to AA a couple of times a week and meeting with a sponsor.

CASE REVISITED: *After our first visit, C was in the contemplation stage because she was willing to consider that there were drawbacks to continuing to use cocaine, but she did not see anything wrong with her marijuana use. At her next visit, we discuss her distress about her anxiety symptoms and problems with her job performance, as well as financial issues. I ask her to tell me about a typical day, including where her drug use fits in. This helps her recognize that the drugs aren't doing much to help with her anxiety symptoms, and that they take time away from other things she wants to accomplish. I ask her to start making a list of the pros and cons of her cocaine use before her next visit.*

At our next visit, C is in the preparation stage regarding her cocaine use, but still in contemplation about her marijuana use. She asks about options to help her cut down on cocaine, although she is not yet ready to commit to beginning a program. I give her options to consider, including going to Narcotics Anonymous meetings, meeting with a therapist for individual counseling, or looking into a residential program covered by her health care insurance. C says she will consider these and discuss them at our next session.

The real value of the Stages of Change model is its reminder that patients are ultimately responsible for their behavior change; as clinicians, all we can do is facilitate the process. This doesn't imply that we passively think, "This person is just stubborn; he'll have to do his own thing and come back to me when he's decided he needs treatment." Instead, as a facilitator, it's our job to try to increase that patient's intrinsic motivation, and to help him recognize the risks of his behavior and the potential options he has.

The Stages of Change model also helps prevent us from becoming frustrated about a patient's lack of progress. Some people simply need more time than we anticipate to make changes. It's important to remember that the patient sets the pace, and that we should always meet patients where they are in the process. If a patient in my care keeps relapsing, I don't bang my head against the wall—instead, I recognize that the patient has fallen back to an earlier stage, and we work through the process again.

Brief intervention: The FRAMES technique

The techniques of MI work very well with brief interventions. Brief intervention's important elements can be summed up with the mnemonic FRAMES: Feedback, Responsibility, Advice, Menu, Empathy, and Self-efficacy (Bien et al, 1993). I suggest you keep this mnemonic in mind during your sessions. Even if you have only a few minutes with a patient, you will always be able to touch on at least one of these interventions.

Feedback. The goal of feedback is to promote awareness of the costs of the present course of behavior in order to motivate your patient to seek treatment. This can include going over abnormal lab results like liver function tests, pointing out evidence of physical tolerance such as escalating doses, connecting legal problems (such as a DUI) or frequent job changes with current drug use, or helping the patient realize that current family problems are a direct result of drinking or drug use. It's also helpful to enlist your patient's spouse and other family members in providing this kind of feedback.

Responsibility. Remind patients that they are ultimately responsible for making the changes needed to improve their life. This involves helping to identify their personal goals for growth—which can help patients see the discrepancy between where they are and where they want to be.

Advice. Provide clear, concrete advice to make a change in drinking or drug use.

Menu. Provide a range of options so that patients can take an active part in the treatment process. I try to stick with two or three options to avoid overwhelming them with choices.

Empathy. Empathy is the basic building block of therapy; don't forget to use it!

Self-efficacy. Self-efficacy is a patient's belief that success at a specific task is possible. You can facilitate this by setting a series of simple, attainable early goals toward recovery that will increase your patient's self-confidence when accomplished.

⬤ **CLINICAL PEARLS: Two Useful MI Techniques**
Here are two techniques that I often use with patients when helping them to discover their motivations for quitting.

1. Good things and less-good things

This is a handy, nonthreatening way to help patients build up their ambivalence about their use.

First, ask them what they like about their drug use—for example, "Tell me some of the good things about your marijuana use." They will enumerate the various positive effects of the drug. Then say, "Are there some things that are less good about it?" As patients think this question through, they often discover that certain aspects of their lives have been damaged or impaired by their substance use.

2. A typical day

This is a particularly good technique for patients who are not talkative. It's also a good general question for beginning your substance use evaluation. Say, "Walk me through a typical day of yours, starting from when you get up."

One unexpected benefit to this technique is in those cases where patients don't mention the drug at all in their description. I'll ask why they haven't, and will often hear about a negative consequence, like, "On a typical day I go to classes, and I can't use when I go." This opens the doors to some self-motivational statements, such as, "Using drugs makes it hard for me to do well in school."

RELAPSE PREVENTION THERAPY

Relapse prevention therapy (RPT) has been shown to be effective for various substance use disorders (see for example Irvin JE et al, *J Consult Clin Psychol* 1999;67(4):563–570). There are formal procedures for this type of therapy, often involving group sessions with structured activities. But the essence of the approach can be applied during short individual visits, and I suggest you budget some time during every meeting to discuss relapse prevention techniques. A good way to open that conversation is by asking questions such as: "Do you see any barriers that would be a problem to your recovery?" "Is there something that could derail the train here?" "What are your concerns and thoughts about abstinence? Are there any challenges?"

The key to relapse prevention is planning ahead. Have patients envision scenarios where they might be tempted to use, like going to a party or walking down a street and meeting their former dealer. Have them talk through their plans for dealing with these kinds of situations. Often, you will help patients develop "refusal skills," which are strategies for successfully turning down opportunities to use substances. You can elicit refusal skills by saying, "Give me some examples of what you could say [or do] in these risky situations. What words would you actually use?"

Example of refusal skills include:

- Saying, "No thank you, I'm not going to use because . . ." Coming up with a list of specific excuses ahead of time helps patients resist peer pressure and harden their resolve.
- Saying, "Not right now" or, "Maybe another time." This is sometimes easier than saying no because these phrases sound less judgmental about the offer.
- Changing the subject.
- Suggesting an alternative activity.

> ⭘ **CLINICAL PEARL: The HALT Reminder**
> *HALT is a well-known mnemonic for some emotional and physical states that can lead to relapse: Hungry, Angry, Lonely, Tired. Encourage patients to recall these when they are tempted to relapse. Often, simply identifying the root of temptation gives them the fortitude to do something to resolve it.*

Common causes of relapse

Some of the most common reasons for relapse are self-medication, temptation, overconfidence, and boredom. I discuss each of these reasons below, along with suggestions for how to help your patients work through them.

Self-medication

Patients recognize that using drugs helps them deal with stress, at least on a temporary basis. It's your job to help them come up with some alternative solutions. For example, I had a patient who said, "My mother-in-law is coming to visit next week, and I always drink more when she's around." My response was to ask what made him drink more when she was visiting. He described some sources of chronic conflict and tension between the two of them. I offered a few commonsense suggestions to offset self-medication, such as:

- Enlisting his spouse's help. "Tell your partner that you're trying not to drink while enduring a visit with a particularly stressful person. The two of you can come up with ways ahead of time to try and defuse some of the tension. Or perhaps your spouse could just give you a simple reminder that your goal is abstinence."
- Avoidance. "Find excuses to attend to some matters in another part of the house or make plans to be out of the house for a while."
- Considering timing. "Perhaps you should delay your quit attempt until after a potentially stressful visit or plan a visit when your sobriety is better established."

Temptation ("because it's there")

When patients expose themselves to temptation, they are asking for trouble. Otherwise known as "triggers," these are situations that make it harder for your patient to abstain. These include going to the bar or even driving by it on the way home, walking through a neighborhood where one is likely to interact with drug dealers, or spending time with certain people who use drugs. I will often have patients write down a list of such triggers and discuss how to avoid them or cope with them successfully. This is sometimes referred to as "avoiding people, places, and things" (that are triggers to use).

For example, a patient's job required him to go to social functions where alcohol was served. He worried that others would notice if he didn't drink and would suspect that he had a drinking problem (he did, but it wasn't something he wanted to advertise!). He would feel self-conscious in these scenarios and sometimes would feel obligated to drink. Some suggestions we discussed included:

- Do some reality testing: "If you didn't have a drink, would this really be such a terrible thing for your job?" "How likely is it that your colleagues are keeping track of what you are ordering?"
- Think of specific excuses or explanations ahead of time (ie, refusal skills)—for example, "I'll tell them my doctor said I shouldn't drink because of heartburn pain."
- Substitute a nonalcoholic beverage and nurse this drink throughout the social function.

FUN FACT: Nonalcoholic Beers

Nonalcoholic beers, by law, can actually contain a small amount of alcohol (0.5% or less). This is why they are also referred to as low-alcohol beer or near-beer. Because they have such a low alcohol content, these drinks can also legally be sold to minors.

Nonalcoholic beer is brewed like regular beer, but before bottling it, there is an extra heating step to remove the alcohol, since alcohol has a lower boiling point than water and will boil off first. The heating process may, however, change the flavor of the beer, which is a common complaint. Websites such as beeradvocate.com have reader reviews from across the spectrum of nonalcoholic beers. So if your patient's main argument against these drinks (besides the obvious) is that "they taste like fizzy yellow water," suggest looking up the reviews and trying some other brands.

Overconfidence

Patients who have been abstinent for a while can become overconfident in their ability to use in a controlled way. They start thinking about the good times and tell themselves, "Using once in a while won't hurt." Unfortunately, this attitude often leads to relapse. You want to find out about patients' rationale and help play up the ambivalence. They may have a romanticized ideal about what life was like when they were using. Carefree use might seem appealing. Remind them that it wasn't all days of wine and roses; there were plenty of consequences that led them to make the change in the first place.

Some patients will rationalize that they can have a few drinks at a particular event, like a wedding or a sports game, and that compartmentalizing their drinking in this way won't lead to relapse. In these instances, I'll ask: "Are there particular reasons why you are having these thoughts of drinking at this point in time?" "Is drinking appealing to you just because of this [wedding, anniversary party, etc], or are you having more cravings?" "Have you been feeling more anxious or depressed about something?"

While I never tell patients that a return to controlled use is out of the question, I will let them know that it's unlikely to work out. I'll say, "In my experience, controlled use doesn't work very well. That has not been an achievable goal for most of my patients."

Boredom

Most patients in recovery realize that they need to stay busy and focused on things, like work, hobbies, and volunteering. I find that folksy metaphors sometimes work well: "The devil finds work for idle hands." Talk about old hobbies that might be worth revisiting now that your patient is feeling healthier and has more free time. Some people feel better when they dive into a new situation or hobby with a group of people unrelated to their former lifestyle choices. And some patients feel rewarded by getting involved in sponsor roles or efforts to support others with substance use issues, though for others this may hit too close to home. Keep a dialogue going about how patients are filling their time.

Advice From Terence Gorski, an Expert on Relapse Prevention

(Adapted from an article written by Terence Gorski for the *Carlat Addiction Treatment Report*, November 2013. Mr. Gorski is the founder and president of The CENAPS Corporation.)

I will often have clients write down their life and addiction history and look at why they relapsed in the past. I will then have them develop a list of early warning signs of impending relapse. These would include things like irrational thoughts and unmanageable feelings, as well as situations, such as hanging around with old drug-using peers, that may lead them back to substance use.

We will then work together to put into place strategies for preventing relapse. These include detailed daily planning and personal check-ins with sponsors, friends, or family members, to make sure they are keeping with the program. I will have clients write a "recovery plan"—a schedule of activities that they know will help them stay sober, such as working a 12-step program and attending relapse prevention support groups—and compare it to the list of high-risk situations and early relapse warning signs. What will clients do when faced with a high-risk situation? Techniques include mental rehearsal, role-playing, and therapeutic assignments. For example, if a client goes into a bar where he used to drink, he will plan to call his AA sponsor and go to the next available AA meeting.

I recommend that clients start each day by reading something that focuses the mind on sober and responsible living and then mindfully planning the day. They should end the day by confirming that they completed everything on the recovery plan and reflecting on how they dealt with various challenges. If there are issues, clients then decide whether to tap into their support network to talk about the day before going to bed.

It's crucial to schedule recovery checkups with clients to review and update the relapse prevention plan. At minimum, I recommend monthly visits for 3 months, quarterly visits for the next 2 years, and then annual visits for at least the next 5 years. (A detailed clinical manual, "Recovery Management Check-Ups: An Early Re-Intervention Approach," is available at http://tinyurl.com/j5bfzu5.)

Journaling for relapse avoidance

I encourage most of my patients to journal, and I emphasize its importance in the recovery process. I keep my instructions simple and say something like, "You need to write a half a page a day, and I want you to bring your notebook to each visit."

There are multiple benefits to journaling:

- Writing things down helps my patients get a clearer sense of how their lives are going.
- I have a better idea of what's running through their heads.
- As time goes on, I can review past entries with patients to demonstrate how much better things are getting.
- Journaling helps alert me to situations we aren't discussing in the office, usually related to relationships—a patient's entries can sometimes reveal an enabler.
- For those in AA, I can discern what they are getting out of the meetings, and what they are learning from the Big Book of AA.

I often write a sentence or two in my notes about what patients put in their journals as a reminder.

CASE CONCLUSION: *After the third visit, C was in preparation. Now, at the fourth visit, she is ready for the action stage. She has thought about the menu of choices I gave her, and decides to start seeing a psychologist for individual counseling. She also decides to set a quit date for cocaine for a couple of weeks later, during a time when she will be under less stress. C is*

able to stop using cocaine, and this accomplishment allows her to eventu-
ally work on stopping her marijuana use.

Self-Test Questions

1. A 45-year-old man is admitted to the hospital with pneumonia. During
   the admission evaluation, he admits to smoking 1 pack of cigarettes per
   day, as well as drinking at least 3 beers daily for the past 10 years, but
   he states he did not think these habits were problematic. The hospital
   physician begins motivational interviewing techniques to enhance the
   patient's readiness to consider changing his behavior regarding drinking
   and smoking. By the time the patient is discharged from the hospital, he
   recognizes that he has a problem with his use of alcohol and tobacco, but
   he is not yet ready to plan on making a quit attempt. At the time of his
   discharge, which stage of change is this patient in?
   a. Action
   b. Contemplation
   c. Maintenance
   d. Pre-contemplation

2. A 30-year-old man comes to the emergency department after experiencing chest pain and blurred vision for the past 3 hours. He admits to
   using a few lines of cocaine every couple of months when he needs to
   work long hours to finish a project. He has 3–4 mixed drinks a few times
   a year. Which of the following is the best method to motivate this patient
   to change his substance use pattern?
   a. Obtain a detailed history of the patient's cocaine use in the past week
   b. Explore the patient's alcohol use in the past month
   c. Explore the connection between the patient's alcohol and cocaine use
   d. Ask the patient to rate his level of readiness to change his cocaine use
      on a scale from 1 to 10

3. A 20-year-old woman is in early recovery from methamphetamine use
   disorder and undergoing individual therapy. Her counselor works with
   her on ways to successfully deal with triggers to use, as well as role-playing what to say and do if she is in a situation where she is tempted to use.
   Which of the following best describes this type of addiction treatment?
   a. Avoiding people, places, and things

   b. Dialectical behavioral therapy

   c. Relapse prevention therapy

   d. Motivational interviewing

The answer key for these self-test questions is on page 233.

Note: If you purchased CME credit with this book, your CME post-test can be accessed when you are logged in at www.thecarlatreport.com/AddictionGuide. Please keep in mind that the question and answer order for that CME post-test are different than what you see in these self-test study questions.

CHAPTER 5

12-Step Programs

**"To this day, I am amazed at how many of my problems—
most of which had nothing to do with drinking, I believed—
have become manageable or have simply disappeared
since I quit drinking."**
Alcoholics Anonymous

TAKE HOME POINTS

- Alcoholics Anonymous (AA) and Narcotics Anonymous (NA) are mutual help organizations based on the Twelve Steps.
- Advise patients to try some meetings; attending 2 to 3 meetings per week is associated with the most benefit.
- Although you don't need to memorize the Twelve Steps, becoming familiar with the basics of AA/NA can help you help your patients.
- Encourage patients to do more than just attend meetings—they should also get a phone list and find a sponsor.
- Advise patients to try several different meetings before giving up on 12-step programs.
- Alternative self-help groups are also available.

CASE VIGNETTE: *E is a 28-year-old woman with a long history of severe alcohol and cannabis use. She began drinking in earnest during college, and has had only brief periods of sobriety since then. She was recently placed on medical leave from her job in order to be admitted to a detox and rehab facility. It's clear that this is her last chance to get sober before she is fired. Her previous psychiatrist had prescribed acamprosate to reduce her cravings and recommends that she attend AA meetings. E responds, "I can't do AA. I tried it, and I can't deal with the religious stuff."*

How would you respond to E's reluctance to attend AA? How valuable is it for severe alcohol users to attend 12-step meetings? What are the steps?

INTRODUCTION: AA'S HISTORY

12-step organizations (AA, NA, and others) are the most commonly sought sources of help for substance-related problems in the U.S. All are considered mutual help organizations (MHOs) and have certain features in common: They are self-supporting, open to anyone with a desire to stop substance use, and do not have professional facilitators.

AA, founded in 1935, is the original and by far the most popular MHO, with more than 50,000 meetings a week nationwide. AA grew out of a Christian organization called the Oxford Group, which was founded in 1931 by Frank Buchman, an American Lutheran minister. Buchman had a religious conversion experience on a trip to England, and in 1921, during a visit to Oxford University, he formed a religious fellowship called A First Century Christian Fellowship. By 1931, its name had changed to the Oxford Group. This group had elements that would later be adopted by AA, including a rejection of hierarchies, an emphasis on beliefs rather than religion, and a specific series of stages to follow in order to improve one's life (mirrored later in AA's Twelve Steps).

The eventual co-founder of AA, William Griffith Wilson, was born in 1895 in East Dorset, Vermont, where his parents ran an inn and tavern. At some point, both of his parents abandoned him, and Wilson was raised by his grandparents. Not surprisingly, he suffered episodes of depression from an early age, and also had significant social anxiety. He discovered alcohol in 1917, and it quickly became his constant companion. Though he went to law school, he did not graduate because he was too drunk to pick up his diploma. A subsequent career as a stock broker also ended in shambles.

When an old drinking buddy, Ebby Thacher, visited him in 1934, Wilson was astonished to find that Thacher had been sober for several weeks. Thacher credited the Oxford Group, which had opened branches in New York City and Akron, Ohio, with helping him gain sobriety through Christian fellowship. With his encouragement, Wilson attended a meeting, but continued drinking and soon thereafter was admitted to a detox hospital, where he went into delirium tremens. During that hospitalization, he had a life-changing religious experience in which he saw a flash of light and felt the presence of God.

Wilson never drank again. The following year, in 1935, he met another alcoholic member of the Oxford Group, a physician named Bob Smith,

> ### FUN FACT: AA and the Bronx Cocktail
> Bill Wilson had his first drink during military training in Massachusetts. He went to a dinner party and drank some Bronx cocktails (which are classic gin martinis with a splash of orange juice). According to *Time* magazine, he recalled that the drinks liberated him from his shyness: "I had found the elixir of life" (Cheever, 1999).

and the two of them formed a sub-group within the Oxford Group that eventually split off to become AA. In 1939, Wilson published *Alcoholics Anonymous*, eventually known as "The Big Book" because of its heft. Still the basic textbook for AA, it is one of the best-selling books of all time, having sold over 30 million copies.

NA was formed as an offshoot of AA in the 1950s and follows the same principles.

Does AA work?

AA has been a fixture of alcoholism treatment for decades. But does it actually work? The question is hard to answer, in part because it's difficult to do a randomized controlled trial of AA. Such a study would have to track whether patients assigned to AA treatment are attending meetings—a difficult proposition since AA, by definition, is anonymous. Another challenge is that AA groups vary in size, content, and focus, making it hard to define the treatment under study.

This doesn't mean that AA can't be studied—just that doing so requires creative methods. One such method was Project MATCH. This was a large randomized trial in which 1,726 alcoholics were randomly assigned to one of three treatments: cognitive behavioral therapy (CBT), motivational enhancement therapy (MET), and a third treatment that was a stand-in for AA: a psychotherapy, based on encouraging AA attendance, called twelve step facilitation (TSF) (Project MATCH Research Group, 1997).

At both one- and three-year follow-ups, all three interventions were equally helpful at reducing the quantity and frequency of alcohol use. However, TSF was superior to CBT and MET at increasing rates of continuous abstinence: 24% of patients in the TSF condition were continuously abstinent at one year after treatment, compared with 15% and 14% in CBT and MET, respectively (Tonigan et al, 2003).

⬤ **CLINICAL PEARL: The Books of AA**

While we often hear about "The Big Book," many clinicians don't understand exactly what it is and how it is used. The Big Book is a thick blue volume, just short of 600 pages. The first edition was written in 1939, and it has been updated periodically since then. In each edition, the first 164 pages are always the same: the original description of the Twelve Steps written by Bill Wilson. The language from the 1930s is old-fashioned and can be difficult to read for many. The remainder of the book consists of short stories about people's journey to recovery that are written in a modern style.

For those seeking to understand the philosophy of AA, many would agree that the better book to read is Twelve Steps and Twelve Traditions *(known informally as "the Twelve and Twelve"), which was originally written in the 1940s but is updated and revised regularly. Clocking in at 192 pages, the Twelve and Twelve is more readable and is recommended for clinicians who want to achieve a better understanding of the organization.*

There are also several brief pamphlets, each only about a dozen pages, that give information about AA. These can be ordered online from www.aa.org to keep in a waiting room for patients, or a single copy can be printed for free as a reference for the clinician. Two pamphlets I use are A Brief History of Alcoholics Anonymous *and* AA as a Resource for the Health Care Professional.

Does Project MATCH prove that AA is effective? Not really, but it shows that if you base a therapy around AA principles and encourage patients to go to meetings, they will probably do at least as well as other well-validated treatments.

A systematic Cochrane review of the best scientific studies on AA and TSF found that they were as effective as any of the interventions to which they were compared for some factors, such as retention in treatment; however, the review found that no studies unequivocally proved AA and TSF were superior to other treatments (Ferri et al, 2006). Other studies have found a linear dose-response relationship between AA attendance and favorable drinking outcomes (Kaskutas, 2009). Attending one meeting per week, on average, appears to be the minimum threshold to realize benefit, and higher meeting frequency is associated with progressively greater rates of abstinence.

Finally, some research has tried to pinpoint the means by which AA works. AA's key ingredients appear to be helping people make positive changes in their social networks (eg, disassociating themselves with heavy drinkers/drug users and increasing ties with abstainers/low-risk drinkers), and enhancing coping skills and self-efficacy for abstinence when encountering high-risk social situations (see, for example, Kelly JF et al, *Drug Alcohol Depend* 2011;114(2–3):119–126).

WHAT ARE THE TWELVE STEPS?

As a psychiatrist, you don't have to memorize all of the Twelve Steps, but you should become familiar with them if you intend to treat patients with substance use disorder. The underlying idea behind the 12-step program is that stopping alcohol or other drug use is only the beginning of a journey. In order to maintain sobriety, alcohol and drugs must be replaced with something just as compelling. The Twelve Steps represent a series of guidelines for how people might choose to live their lives without alcohol.

Because the steps can be confusing for those not in the program, here is a good way to remember the gist. There are three phases: surrendering, confessing, and maintaining. Steps 1–3 involve realizing that substances have rendered life unmanageable, and that the way out is to surrender to the program (sometimes conceptualized as God in AA literature). Steps 4–9 are a process of listing one's "bad" deeds and confessing them. Steps 10–12 describe how one can best maintain a commitment to sobriety. (See the table at the end of the chapter for a concise list of the twelve steps.)

[Editor's note: The material in the following section was adapted from the article by Alison Knopf, "The Twelve Steps Explained," that appeared in the *Carlat Addiction Treatment Report*, November/December 2015.]

Step 1: The surrender: "We admitted we were powerless over alcohol—that our lives had become unmanageable."

Patients understand that repeated attempts to cut down or stop drinking have not worked—in other words, they have been "powerless." In addition, they understand that there is a connection between drinking and what has brought them to treatment, such as financial problems, job loss, family problems, arrest, or feeling sick—that is the "unmanageable" piece. The sense of relief that comes with the admission of powerlessness and unmanageability in terms of alcohol is liberating for many.

Step 2: The higher power: "Came to believe that a Power greater than ourselves could restore us to sanity."

Many patients who go to AA talk about a "spiritual awakening" that often occurs very early in recovery. That awakening is often a result of Step 2. While going to AA meetings, patients become engaged in the process of recovery, sometimes for the first time. The act of going to the meetings, and of speaking in a supportive setting, gives patients the feeling of taking the initiative. It also inspires a sense of hope, which can be experienced so intensely as to seem religious or spiritual.

Step 3: The decision: "Made a decision to turn our will and our lives over to the care of God as we understood Him."

This step is really just an extension of Step 2, which was about believing in a higher power; this step says explicitly that the patients will trust that higher power. Many members will substitute other terms or concepts for God, such as spirit, nature, the AA process, or the support of AA members.

Step 4: The self-assessment: "Made a searching and fearless moral inventory of ourselves."

In some ways, Step 4 is the crux of AA. It entails writing down (or typing out) the list of behaviors and negative emotions that have caused patients shame over the years. For example, "I told my wife that I would stop drinking but continued to drink, hiding bottles of vodka in the garbage shed. I would say I was taking out the garbage in order to take a few swigs." Unresolved guilt tends to fester and often helps drive people to continue drinking. The therapeutic value of this step lies in patients' strengthened insight into what spurs their drinking, and in preparing for Step 5.

Step 5: The sponsor (or psychiatrist): "Admitted to God, to ourselves, and to another human being the exact nature of our wrongs."

This is a natural extension of Step 4, and entails verbalizing the written inventory, usually to a sponsor. This may take a couple of hours or a couple of days, as patients read from the list and talk about the feelings that are generated. The sponsor has lived through a similar litany of events and is completely nonjudgmental. Therapeutically, this step reduces shame and guilt. A common AA expression is, "We are as sick as our secrets."

Step 6: Readiness to change: "Were entirely ready to have God remove all these defects of character."

Patients have done their self-assessment (Step 4, the moral inventory), and they've shared it with someone (Step 5). With Step 6, it's time for patients to accept that they need to take action to resolve their problems and address any character defects. This is a very short step, something that patients do by themselves. It is a kind of quiet meditation or affirmation of one's readiness to make changes.

Step 7: Humility: "Humbly asked Him to remove our shortcomings."

This is similar to and closely tied to Step 6, with an emphasis on humility and a commitment to use the AA process to stop whatever behaviors led to drinking.

Step 8: Taking responsibility: "Made a list of all persons we had harmed, and became willing to make amends to them all."

AA members often say there are lots of side effects to being an addict. These side effects include the damage done to other people as a result of an addiction. In this step, which is a natural prelude to Step 9, patients make a list of people whom they have harmed, and also list whether they feel harmed by those people. This process helps patients achieve peace of mind, which is another goal of Step 8. Forgiveness of perceived harms is required so that honest amends can be made in the next step.

Step 9: Restitution and amends: "Made direct amends to such people wherever possible, except when to do so would injure them or others."

Whenever possible, patients should make direct amends in order to achieve peace of mind. It is okay to take some time to determine the best way to make amends to a particular individual. Making amends also includes paying—or promising to pay—whatever financial or other obligations are necessary. If a particular form of making amends would harm another person or the patient further, it should generally not be done. However, some members have confessed to crimes as part of Step 9. For example, one member had hit and killed a bicyclist while driving drunk, and left the scene. After long discussions with his sponsor, it was clear that he would not be able to achieve calmness or inner peace until he admitted to the crime. He did so, and served five years in prison—and did not regret that decision.

Step 10: Balance: "Continued to take personal inventory and when we were wrong promptly admitted it."

Step 10 means patients put aside some time at the beginning or end of each day to reflect on their recent behaviors and to judge whether those behaviors have been in alignment with their values. It's a kind of self-regulation that seeks to ensure any new problems will be corrected quickly.

Step 11: Connectedness: "Sought through prayer and meditation to improve our conscious contact with God as we understood Him, praying only for knowledge of His will for us and the power to carry that out."

AA members try to maintain a sense of connection to something outside of themselves. This step often entails some type of meditation or reflection about patients' place in the world. The point is to have some regular form of emotional balance-keeping, such as meditation or daily reflective walks. This step helps patients' awareness of themselves and improves well-being.

Step 12: Helping others: "Having had a spiritual awakening as the result of these steps, we tried to carry this message to alcoholics, and to practice these principles in all our affairs."

Part of continuing recovery for patients—usually former patients by this point—includes helping other alcoholics. This might entail becoming a sponsor, but according to AA philosophy, the best way to help others is to embody AA's principles in one's own life, which will naturally attract other alcoholics to a different way of living. Helping others is a unique aspect of mutual support groups based on the Twelve Steps.

The Twelve Traditions: AA's instruction manual

Aside from the Twelve Steps, AA also has the "Twelve Traditions." These are less well-known, but constitute a sort of manual for how meetings should operate. For example, one tradition involves eligibility: The only requirement for AA membership, which means attending meetings, is "a desire to stop drinking." All AA groups must be self-supporting, can collect donations from members but nobody else, and must not own any property. Money, according to AA tradition, just distracts from the primary purpose—"helping alcoholics achieve sobriety." Another tradition is that AA doesn't take any positions on anything. Finally, AA members are supposed to be anonymous and not disclose their membership to the media. This is not the same as disclosing that they are in recovery.

CASE REVISITED: *E is reluctant to go to AA meetings because of what she had heard from some other people, even though she has never been to a meeting herself. I inform her that there are many types of AA* *meetings—including nonreligious meetings—and that she should keep an open mind. I encourage her to try 2 or 3 meetings before deciding AA is not for her. She agrees to try attending a couple of meetings, and we look online for some near her home.*

AA MEETINGS: HOW THEY WORK

AA meetings are held in churches, community centers, hospitals, and similar settings. There are many meeting options in most cities, and the best way to find them is through the AA website. Entering a ZIP code will retrieve a list of meetings with dates, times, and, importantly, characteristics of available groups. There are also online meetings.

Here are some examples of meeting types:

- Open meetings (anyone may attend) vs. closed meetings (only substance users may attend)
- Alcohol-focused vs. polysubstance abuse
- Gender-specific meetings (women only)
- Older people (eg, "Gray AA")
- Christian-based
- Special professional groups, such as "caduceus meetings" for health care professionals and "birds of a feather" for airline pilots
- Groups that focus on a reading from a book or a pamphlet

Beyond these categories, different meetings tend to attract people of different socioeconomic groups, varying degrees of religiosity, etc. I emphasize to my patients that if they don't like the first meeting they attend, they may be able to find a different meeting where they feel more comfortable. I'll sometimes use the analogy of drinking: "The first time you went to a bar, if you didn't feel comfortable, you didn't say, 'Well, I'm not going to drink at all.' Instead, you went to another bar. AA is a little like that."

People are allowed to come to meetings drunk, as long as they are not disruptive—the only requirement is a desire to quit. While I certainly don't encourage combining drinking with AA attendance, people have found that they can benefit from meetings under any circumstance. Patients have told me, "Every hour I spend in a meeting is an hour I'm not drinking or using."

AA groups often have a steering committee of members who make decisions about how their meetings will be organized. Various officers are elected, such as a treasurer and a secretary, who run the meetings.

Depending on the steering group's decision, most meetings take one of three forms:

1. Speaker meetings. A speaker, usually a member of the group, is invited to tell his or her story of recovery. The floor is then opened for questions or comments. Members often find their sponsors by approaching speakers whose stories are similar to their own.

2. Topic meetings. These meetings are organized around a particular topic, such as coping with the holidays, the place of gratitude in people's lives, or dealing with road rage. Sometimes the topic is a particular AA step, in which case they are called "step meetings."

3. Reading meetings. Such meetings begin with a reading from the library of AA literature, such as The Big Book, and proceed to a discussion of issues raised.

AA meetings usually last about an hour. People gradually arrive, and there is some pre-meeting chitchat, snacking, and coffee drinking. Then the secretary will start the meeting, often with the serenity prayer: "God grant me the courage to change the things I can change, the serenity to accept the things I can't change, and the wisdom to know the difference."

CLINICAL PEARL: Attending an AA Meeting
I highly recommend that you go to at least one AA meeting. It's a moving experience that reminds us why we are doing our work with clients.

Meetings are quite welcoming to new members. Often, someone will ask, "Anyone here for the first time?" First-timers will raise their hands (which is optional) and introduce themselves, usually with the standard, "Hi, my name is Michael, and I'm an alcoholic." Everyone responds, "Hi, Michael." (AA is on a first-name basis only, and members don't even have to use their real names.) As a health professional attending an open meeting, you might say something like, "I'm Michael, and I'm a local treatment professional here to see what this group is like. I'm thinking of recommending it to my clients."

After these opening rituals, the meeting proper will get underway. For example, in a step meeting, the secretary might say, "Today we are going to look at Step 4—everyone get out your Big Book." There might be a reading from the book, and then someone might stand up and say, "Here's how I've dealt with Step 4," and share something about how they made amends. The floor might then be opened for anybody to stand up and respond to the speaker, or to share something unrelated.

How AA sponsorship works

A key element of AA is the networking that occurs between meetings. Patients who benefit the most are those who participate actively in the meetings, but also those who connect with other members, which is how they find a sponsor. The process of finding a sponsor is often gradual. Clients might start by getting together a "phone list," which includes a few people they are comfortable with who are willing to make themselves available to talk. Some groups have a list of people who have volunteered to serve that purpose.

We hear a lot about the importance of sponsors in a patient's recovery. Sponsors must have at least 2 years of solid recovery and have worked through the Twelve Steps completely. They are comfortable and willing to pass on some of their hard-won wisdom to newer members. They may have tools to share, such as 12-step workbooks and worksheets. Clients will have regular contact with a sponsor, though the specific frequency will vary. Some sponsors will say, "Call or text me once a day to see how you're doing." Others will say, "We'll get together after the meeting each week and go to a diner and talk, or work through the steps." It's fine to work with a sponsor "candidate" to see how comfortable the relationship is. Sponsors should generally be the same gender as the member in order to ensure the focus stays on working the steps.

CASE REVISITED: *During recovery, E gets to know a few of the people she continually sees at meetings, so she obtains their phone numbers and calls them periodically. After a while, she gets to know a woman close to her age who has been in recovery for nearly 15 years; she asks this woman to be her sponsor.*

Working with patients as they attend meetings

Other than attending a meeting to understand what it's like, I don't think it's beneficial for a therapist to get involved in continual meeting attendance, beyond asking clients whether they are going to meetings. By the time patients have gone to a few meetings, they'll know more about the process than you do. Once you start talking about the steps in detail, this knowledge gap can be damaging. For example, most first-timers find the first of the Twelve Steps very scary—they're telling people what they are ashamed of. Use a lot of discretion when broaching this subject and a disclaimer about how little you know.

As a psychiatrist doing relatively brief medication-focused visits, you won't have the time to discuss 12-step meetings in great depth, but there are various questions that you can ask your patient during the appointment to reinforce meaningful participation:

- "How often are you attending meetings?" For those with severe alcohol use, attending a minimum of 2 to 3 meetings per week is optimal. If patients have only been to one meeting and didn't like it, ask them about the experience. This will not only help you figure out what sort of meeting might be a better fit, but also may be useful in helping another patient. You should have a few meetings that you think are appropriate to refer patients to. Avoid meetings that are too hardline, or where the members are too domineering. I tend to steer patients who are new to AA to larger meetings to help them feel less self-conscious.

- "Have you gotten your phone list together? Have you thought about looking for a sponsor?" I ask these questions during follow-up visits. If patients haven't assembled their list, probe a bit: "Why not? Have you not been staying after the meeting?" You want to establish that they are interacting with someone individually, someone they can work the steps with outside of the meetings, rather than just with the general group. Research has found that individual involvement is more strongly associated with drinking outcomes than meeting attendance alone (Krentzman et al, 2013).

- "What step are you working on?" While you don't want to take on the role of a sponsor, you should be familiar enough with the Twelve Steps to discuss them with your patients, at least at a superficial level. This is helpful for treatment, and if a patient rejects AA after a couple meetings, you can often use an understanding of the steps to reinforce further attendance.

Unless you have substantial experience with the Twelve Steps, either because you have been treating addictions or because you have worked the program yourself, I don't recommend getting into detailed discussions of the steps with your patients. For those who do have some experience, here are some of the issues that often come up.

Step 1, powerlessness and unmanageability. Some criticize the first step as undermining the individual's self-empowerment. But in my view, it is in sync with the DSM-5 criteria for alcohol use disorder, which include a loss of control ("powerlessness") over one's alcohol use in the face of very negative effects on relationships, work, and other aspects of life ("unmanageability"). I might say, "Step 1 doesn't mean that you are unable to address your problem or have no responsibility for it. As a matter of fact, it's quite the opposite; the steps are about you taking responsibility for your own recovery and moving forward."

Understanding this step can also be helpful for patients who are having trouble with cravings and are on the brink of relapse. I often say something like, "Let's just take a look at the first step again and your recognition of the powerlessness and unmanageability of the disease." That helps to remind patients of the consequences of using. Of course, for any patients who feel close to relapsing, it can be helpful to encourage them to go to an AA meeting and share with the group that they feel like drinking. In AA, this response is viewed as an act of courage and strength rather than weakness—it is normal for an alcoholic to feel like drinking. Assure patients that they will receive a great deal of support from the AA group following such an admission.

Step 2, the higher power. Patients may express discomfort with the idea of a higher power, especially those who are not interested in religion. I emphasize that there are many ways to conceive of the higher power. Some people, indeed, think of it as a Christian god. For others, it's the group dynamic itself. One group literally had a box on a shelf with "higher power" written on it. Another group said that the higher power was the light bulb in the room, something that provides light and facilitates important conversations at meetings. One person told me he viewed it as the ocean, because it is large and powerful and all-surrounding. In AA it is defined as "God as we understand Him," which allows a lot of latitude.

Step 4, the moral inventory. Doing a moral inventory is difficult because it means looking at negative events of an individual's life. This can contribute to depression, and some people get stuck on this step and feel worse and worse. One way to facilitate this step is to say, "So, it's great that you're on the fourth step; when are you planning to complete it?" You could also say, "It may be beneficial if you set a date for the fifth step (where the inventory is shared with another person), carry this out and get it over with, and move on to the other steps." It's important to point out that identifying one's strengths can also be a part of the fourth step's inventory.

Step 9, making amends. Making amends can take time to carry out. Family relationships in particular can be tricky for patients who are adult children of alcoholics, who were molested as children, or whose harmed relatives are now deceased. In those cases, attempts to make amends may harm the other person or simply be unfeasible, and you can point out these issues to your patients.

Steps 10, 11, 12, maintenance steps. When patients are tempted to use again, I emphasize the last three steps, which are considered maintenance steps— meant to be continued throughout a person's life on a regular basis. Ask, "Are you using the 10th, 11th, and 12th steps on a daily basis?" (Some people in 12-step meetings call them "daily disciplines.") "What are you doing daily to support your recovery?" "You've stayed sober today; how did you accomplish that?" Some people will say, "I attend a meeting every day" or, "I call someone in AA everyday just to check in and discuss things." Some people use prayer or meditation. Others do a daily reading from one of the AA textbooks. Regardless of the exact ritual, the key is consistency, and you can emphasize the importance of this practice.

Potential barriers to AA attendance

Research has shown that you can increase patients' chance of attending a meeting by introducing them to other patients in recovery who are AA members and would be willing to accompany them to a local AA meeting. You can accomplish this by asking for an experienced patient's consent to be contacted by patients who are new to AA.

Here are some potential barriers that clients may bring up:
• "What if someone recognizes me?" Some patients are worried about see-ing someone they know at a meeting. I point out that the group is called Alcoholics Anonymous for a reason—participants promise to maintain confidentiality. I note, "If someone recognizes you, that also means you

recognize them, so it's a standoff." I also say, "You may be surprised at who you end up seeing at a meeting!"

- "I don't have a ride." There is an easy answer to that: "If you can get to the first meeting, you can get to any meeting." People at AA are there to help one another, and helping new members get to meetings is one of the more common forms of mutual self-help. If patients are having a hard time arranging transportation to their first meeting, suggest that they call the local AA central office, which will be able to arrange a ride.
- "What if they find out I'm on medication?" It is true that in the past, AA disapproved of members taking medication, but that attitude is now quite rare. Some older groups may still be militant about not using anything other than the program to quit, but in general, prescribed medications for psychiatric conditions are now accepted, and in fact the majority of meeting attendants are likely taking some medication. There may be more resistance to medication-assisted treatment, such as methadone for opioid use disorder. If patients are nervous about this issue, I might advise a "don't ask, don't tell" approach.

ALTERNATIVES TO AA

Some people will not go to AA meetings, perhaps because of the religious-sounding ideology or some other aspect of the culture that rubs them the wrong way. There are several alternative mutual self-help groups that may appeal to those who have ruled out AA.

- Secular Organization for Sobriety (SOS) is an MHO without the religious overtones of AA. Instead of 12 steps, there are 9 principles, although there is some overlap with the Twelve Steps and Twelve Traditions of AA and NA. More information can be found at www.sossobriety.org.
- SMART Recovery (SMART stands for Self-Management and Recovery Training) is a 4-point program that emphasizes cognitive behavioral techniques. See their website at www.smartrecovery.org.
- Celebrate Recovery is a 12-step group that embraces and incorporates Christian religious teachings into the traditional Twelve Steps. Their website is www.celebraterecovery.com.

Al-Anon and Nar-Anon

Al-Anon is a meeting to support family (or anyone who cares about a person with an alcohol use disorder) of AA members, while Nar-Anon is for

The Twelve Steps: A Quick Reference

Step 1: The surrender: "We admitted we were powerless over alcohol—that our lives had become unmanageable."

Step 2: The higher power: "Came to believe that a Power greater than ourselves could restore us to sanity."

Step 3: The decision: "Made a decision to turn our will and our lives over to the care of God as we understood Him."

Step 4: The self-assessment: "Made a searching and fearless moral inventory of ourselves."

Step 5: The sponsor (or psychiatrist): "Admitted to God, to ourselves, and to another human being the exact nature of our wrongs."

Step 6: Readiness to change: "Were entirely ready to have God remove all these defects of character."

Step 7: Humility: "Humbly asked Him to remove our shortcomings."

Step 8: Taking responsibility: "Made a list of all persons we had harmed, and became willing to make amends to them all."

Step 9: Restitution and amends: "Made direct amends to such people wherever possible, except when to do so would injure them or others."

Step 10: Balance: "Continued to take personal inventory and when we were wrong promptly admitted it."

Step 11: Connectedness: "Sought through prayer and meditation to improve our conscious contact with God as we understood Him, praying only for knowledge of His will for us and the power to carry that out."

Step 12: Helping others: "Having had a spiritual awakening as the result of these steps, we tried to carry this message to alcoholics, and to practice these principles in all our affairs."

family and loved ones of NA members. Like AA, these meetings are free and open to the public, and are often held in the same building as AA meetings. Family members will learn how to be helpful for addicted loved ones without enabling their behavior. Research has shown sustained attendance at Al-Anon benefits families through improved quality of life, increased self-esteem, and decreased depression (Timko et al, 2015).

I've found that Al-Anon is quite helpful, and if I have any interaction with the family, I'll always ask if they are familiar with Al-Anon or Nar-Anon and encourage attendance. Even if the user is not interested in recovery, these meetings are helpful.

CASE CONCLUSION: *After working through the Twelve Steps with her sponsor, E is able to establish her long-term recovery because she gained the support and the coping skills to be successful. She continues going to meetings once or twice a week, and volunteers to be on the designated phone list for her AA group. She enjoys being able to help people who reach out to her, and she looks forward to continuing to work on Step 12 as a sponsor herself in the future.*

Self-Test Questions

1. A 26-year-old man had been using cannabis regularly, but became concerned when it started to interfere with his job performance. He has begun attending Narcotics Anonymous meetings and is starting to look for a sponsor. For this man, which of the following characteristics is most desirable in a prospective sponsor?
   a. Abused the same drug (cannabis)
   b. Clean for 6 months
   c. Opposite sex
   d. Stable in recovery

2. A 39-year-old woman has a long history of problems due to heavy use of alcohol and marijuana, including a history of major depression. She recently achieved abstinence and now attends 12-step meetings at least twice every week. She has become active in a local church doing charity work. Which of the following factors is most important to her continuing abstinence?
   a. Duration of previous alcohol and drug use
   b. Female gender
   c. Frequency of 12-step meeting attendance
   d. Involvement in faith community

3. Which of the following is one of the Twelve Traditions of Alcoholics Anonymous?

a. The only requirement for membership is a desire to stop drinking
b. Membership dues are assessed on an annual basis
c. The group's public relations policy is based on press, radio, and film promotion
d. Individual groups may accept outside contributions

The answer key for these self-test questions is on page 233.

Note: If you purchased CME credit with this book, your CME post-test can be accessed when you are logged in at www.thecarlatreport.com/AddictionGuide. Please keep in mind that the question and answer order for that CME post-test are different than what you see in these self-test study questions.

CHAPTER 6

Dual Diagnosis

"Sometimes we motivate ourselves by thinking of what
we want to become. Sometimes we motivate ourselves
by thinking about who we don't ever want to be again."
Shane Niemeyer

TAKE HOME POINTS

- Try to assess the time course of the substance use disorder vs. the psychiatric disorder.
- Determine whether one disorder is clearly primary, or whether they are co-occurring with no clear primary disorder.
- In most cases, treat both disorders at once.
- It is often helpful to order a urine drug screen to see whether other substances are involved.
- Come up with some strategies for treating anxiety issues in substance users.

CASE VIGNETTE: *You are referred K, a 26-year-old man recently discharged from the local psychiatric hospital. He had been admitted with suicidal ideation to jump in front of a train; at the time, he was on a drinking binge. The discharge summary states that when admitted, he was depressed, suicidal, and intoxicated. Over the course of the admission, he was rapidly detoxed with Librium; after 3 days, he denied suicidal ideation but still felt depressed. K was not prescribed antidepressants because the staff felt that his primary problem was alcohol abuse, and that his depression would likely resolve once he had gained stable sobriety.*

INTRODUCTION

Dual diagnosis is common. Among patients who come to your office with psychiatric issues, at least 20%–50% will also have a substance use issue, with the rate highest in schizophrenia (Regier et al, 1990).

In addition to the case vignette above, here are a couple of other dual diagnosis conundrums that you are likely to encounter:

- A patient with long-standing generalized anxiety disorder (GAD) asks you for a prescription for Adderall, saying she tried some of her son's Adderall and believes she has ADHD like him. You are concerned that she may be abusing the Adderall, and that if you were to prescribe it for her, her anxiety would worsen.

- A patient with a long history of on-again, off-again alcohol use disorder complains of significant panic attacks. He is on SSRIs for depression, and he is asking for a prescription for Klonopin, which "worked before" when he obtained it from another doctor. You are reluctant to prescribe a benzodiazepine to a person with alcohol issues.

How should you approach these types of "messy" patients who have more going on than pure substance use issues? I'll start by outlining my approach to assessing patients with co-occurring disorders, then move on to specific diagnoses and substances. Finally, I'll cover the practical issue of deciding when it's okay to prescribe controlled drugs to patients with substance use disorders.

ASSESSING CO-OCCURRING DISORDERS

CASE REVISITED: *During your evaluation of K, he describes a lifelong sense of low self-esteem, with episodes of depression associated with drinking. He says he binge drinks every few months, and each time he feels sad and ashamed both before and after the episode. After your evaluation, you feel certain that K's drinking episodes and depressed mood are related, but you are not clear whether he drinks because he gets depressed, or whether he becomes depressed because of shame after drinking.*

Which came first: the chicken or the egg? The substance abuse or the psychiatric syndrome?

My approach is to try to get a thorough history of when patients' different problems started. Did they start using drugs in their early teens, then later develop symptoms? If so, I consider the substance use the primary disorder. In other cases, patients describe mood and anxiety symptoms starting at a young age, and recall that they started using substances to deal with the emotional pain—in such a situation, the psychiatric syndrome is primary. Finally, a third possibility is that the two disorders are co-occurring and independent of one another.

A common approach to patients with dual diagnoses is to wait for several weeks of sobriety before deciding whether to treat the co-occurring psychiatric disorder. The idea here is that the substance use muddies the diagnostic picture too much, and rather than start a medication before you are completely certain of the diagnosis, it's better to wait for the actual diagnosis to uncover itself.

While there is some wisdom to this approach, I don't recommend waiting too long before making a diagnosis and treating. For example, one meta-analysis found that it only takes about a week after abstinence to be able to reliably diagnose major depression (Nunes & Levin, 2004). Regardless of which disorder came first, it's better to address both problems early on. For example, in the case of K, I would offer a trial of an antidepressant if his depressive symptoms lasted for a week after sobriety. Offering treatment for the immediate cause of suffering is generally the best thing to do, for a couple reasons: There's a good chance that the patient will feel better sooner, and you will get the patient engaged in treatment right away, strengthening the alliance and, in K's case, increasing the likelihood that he will seek specific treatment for the alcohol use as well.

SPECIFIC PSYCHIATRIC DISORDERS AND SUBSTANCE ISSUES

Dual diagnosis is a large topic, and we don't have room to comprehensively cover it here. Below, I've hit on some of the more common ways in which I have seen substance use and psychiatric disorders interacting.

Bipolar disorder

Stimulant abuse may cause and be confused with mania, though once the effects of the drug wear off, you can usually figure out the true diagnosis. Conversely, mania causes impulsivity that can lead patients to abuse a variety of substances.

> ⭕ **CLINICAL PEARL: Explaining Dual Diagnosis**
> *When treating a patient with dual diagnosis, make a point of explaining that substance use can aggravate or even cause psychiatric issues. While this may seem obvious, in my experience, patients may not recognize the link between the two. They may think the substance helps, even if only temporarily—this may often be true, but it is a poor long-term solution.*

Depression

Alcohol can contribute to depression in a number of ways, both directly and indirectly:

- Alcohol can cause some people to feel euphoria, but others may become angry, depressed, or just withdrawn.
- Although people often believe drinking helps with insomnia, in fact it disrupts sleep architecture, making it hard to achieve restorative sleep. This can aggravate depression.
- Alcohol weakens inhibitions, leading people to make bad choices, which can also worsen depression.
- Some use alcohol as a coping mechanism for difficult situations. While this can be temporarily helpful, it also means patients are not learning how to deal with stress and are not developing good coping skills. Such patients often benefit if you refer them to therapists who are well-versed in coping skill enhancement techniques.

Other substances can contribute to depression as well. Stimulant abusers can crash heavily, leading to anhedonia, irritability, and acute depression. They may have passive suicidal thoughts, though in my experience they rarely become actively suicidal during a crash. Long-term stimulant use can also lead to dopamine depletion, which can bring about long-term depression.

A protracted abstinence syndrome can occur after stopping long-term use of alcohol, sedatives, stimulants, or opioids. The typical scenario is that a patient will go through detox and get over the worst of withdrawal quickly, but notice mood and concentration problems over the ensuing weeks, which can look very much like dysthymia. Thankfully, you can give patients hope by explaining that this is a time-limited problem. I say things like, "You've been altering your neurochemistry with chemicals for years, so it's going to take a while for your brain to reboot. Your brain is slowly healing and returning to the way it was." I encourage patients to resist the temptation to relapse, because they will lose all their gains if they do. The high rate of relapse in the early post-detox period is the reason why Alcoholics Anonymous recommends "90 meetings in 90 days."

When patients are having significant depressive symptoms as a result of prolonged abstinence, antidepressant treatment is effective and recommended.

Anxiety disorders

Many patients use alcohol to reduce anxiety. While effective, alcohol is a very short-acting sedative and requires re-dosing regularly. Alcohol withdrawal increases anxiety and causes a vicious cycle of increased drinking, increased tolerance, and more withdrawal symptoms.

A variety of drugs can cause anxiety directly:
- Stimulants cause paranoia and hypervigilance, especially if used chronically.
- Marijuana can cause paranoia and panic attacks.
- Hallucinogens can cause bad trips, which are basically prolonged panic attacks. PCP (phencyclidine) is particularly notorious for bad trips.

Psychotic disorders

Substance use is nearly universal in patients with schizophrenia and other psychotic disorders. Patients with schizophrenia smoke tobacco at higher rates than the general public. This is particularly problematic because these patients have high rates of metabolic syndrome, and adding smoking to the mix increases the risk of heart disease. Unfortunately, it can be very difficult to get such patients to decrease their smoking. One reason these patients smoke tobacco is that it induces the metabolism of antipsychotic drugs and therefore reduces the severity of side effects.

Hallucinogens cause transient hallucinations, but the real danger is that they can unmask an underlying psychotic disorder. However, they do not cause psychotic disorders in people who would not otherwise develop them. Stimulants can cause paranoid delusions when used chronically, and this can be very hard to distinguish from a primary psychotic disorder. Early onset of marijuana use, as well as frequent use, is associated with first onset of psychotic breaks. Having a family history of psychotic disorder increases this risk.

Neurocognitive disorders

Chronic alcohol use can lead directly to dementia. But even the acute effects of alcohol can be problematic in patients with dementia of other causes, because of its amnestic effects. If a patient is complaining of memory problems and drinking semi-regularly, recommend a trial of abstinence—improvements can be subtle but real. Benzodiazepines can also cause long-term cognitive impairment.

TREATING ANXIETY IN SUBSTANCE ABUSERS

Given how common substance abuse is in psychiatric patients, we are often confronted with the tricky decision about prescribing potentially abusable drugs to substance users (see Table 6-1). In making these decisions, I try

TABLE 6-1. Potential Antianxiety Medications for Substance-Abusing Patients

Medication	FDA-Approved Indications	Mechanism	Recommended Daily Dosage (for SSRIs and SNRIs, representative meds are listed)
SSRIs	Varies with medication; includes depression, GAD, OCD, panic disorder, social anxiety disorder, PTSD, and others	Serotonin reuptake inhibitor	Paroxetine: 20 mg–60 mg Sertraline: 50 mg–200 mg Escitalopram: 10 mg–20 mg
SNRIs	Varies with medication; includes depression, GAD, OCD, panic disorder, social anxiety disorder, PTSD, and others	Serotonin and norepinephrine reuptake inhibitor	Duloxetine: 40 mg–120 mg Venlafaxine XR: 75 mg–225 mg
Buspirone	GAD	Serotonin 5HT1A receptor partial agonist	30 mg–60 mg
Hydroxyzine (Atarax, Vistaril)	"Symptomatic relief of anxiety and tension associated with psychoneurosis" (1956 terminology)	Antihistamine	25 mg–100 mg
Pregabalin (Lyrica)	Post-herpetic neuropathy, diabetic neuropathy, fibromyalgia (GAD in Europe but not in U.S.)	Possible: gamma-aminobutyric acid (GABA) reuptake inhibitor	100 mg–600 mg
Gabapentin (Neurontin)	Epilepsy, post-herpetic neuralgia, restless leg syndrome	Possible: Modulator of GABA	300 mg–900 mg
Quetiapine (Seroquel)	Schizophrenia, bipolar disorder; major depression as adjunct	Dopamine D2 and serotonin 5HT2A antagonist	50 mg–800 mg
Natural medications (valerian)	Not FDA-approved	Possible: Modulator of GABA	200 mg–450 mg in the morning

to estimate how likely it is that a given patient will misuse a drug, either by abusing it or by giving or selling it to someone else. I balance that estimate with the drug's potential benefit for the patient.

A particularly common scenario is the patient with a history of substance abuse who suffers anxiety and is requesting benzodiazepines. While benzodiazepines are effective antianxiety workhorses for many patients, most guidelines tell us to avoid prescribing them to substance abusers. The concerns are that the benzo high will remind patients of their substances of choice, and that benzo withdrawal symptoms will lead to old substance-abusing habits. However, one review of the literature concluded that benzos can safely be prescribed for some alcoholics in recovery (Lingford-Hughes et al, 2002), and most psychiatrists can manage such patients by making sure that they do not escalate their doses and do not get early refills.

Psychotherapy is always an option, and it can work well. For example, a two-week pilot trial of cognitive behavioral therapy–based integrated treatment for panic disorder and alcohol abuse in 48 patients showed benefit over alcoholism treatment alone (Kushner et al, 2006). But assuming therapy has already been tried, what are some reasonable non-benzo approaches?

SSRIs/SNRIs and other antidepressants

Most substance abusers with anxiety will end up rotating through several SSRIs and SNRIs. These are robustly effective medications with few side effects, and we all have our own "go to" meds. Paroxetine carries the most FDA-approved indications for disorders on the anxiety spectrum, but it also is the most likely to cause sexual dysfunction, weight gain, and sedation. Sertraline and escitalopram are good choices in terms of minimal side effects and few drug/drug interactions. The SNRIs, especially duloxetine and levomilnacipran, may be especially appropriate if your patient has a comorbid chronic pain condition, because both of these meds carry FDA indications for pain syndromes. The newer antidepressant vilazodone was effective for GAD in one placebo-controlled trial (Gommoll et al, 2015). You might also consider mirtazapine (Remeron), effective in a small open-label study of GAD and also helpful for insomnia. Bupropion, while not effective for anxiety disorders per se, is effective for anxiety when it is a symptom of depression—but watch out for its common early side effects of insomnia and jitteriness, and note that it is contraindicated in patients withdrawing from alcohol or other sedatives.

Buspirone

Buspirone has been around a long time, and many of your patients will say they've already tried it. Maybe they have, maybe they haven't. Here are two tips to optimize patient response. First, don't oversell it as a benzodiazepine substitute—it doesn't work as quickly or as well, and patients expecting the benzo feeling will be disappointed and stop taking it. Second, get the dose high enough to be effective before throwing in the towel. A robust dose is 60 mg a day, split up either twice or three times daily. Dizziness and sedation may limit the dose.

Hydroxyzine (Atarax, Vistaril)

Some are surprised to hear that hydroxyzine has an FDA indication for anxiety (albeit an old one). It is effective—for example, in one large randomized placebo-controlled trial, patients with GAD randomly assigned to hydroxyzine 50 mg/day did just as well as those assigned to bromazepam 6 mg/day (bromazepam is a benzodiazepine approved in Europe; 6 mg is equivalent to about 10 mg of diazepam). Patients on the benzodiazepine experienced more sedation (Llorca et al, 2002).

Pregabalin (Lyrica)

Pregabalin is a Schedule V controlled substance (the same category as cough suppressants with codeine), so it might seem an odd choice for treating anxiety in patients with substance abuse histories. Wouldn't it pour fuel on the fire? Apparently not. In fact, pregabalin has been compared with naltrexone as a treatment for alcohol dependence; in one small randomized controlled trial, pregabalin was as effective as naltrexone and led to greater improvement in anxiety (Martinotti et al, 2010). Pregabalin's efficacy for GAD (in the absence of substance abuse) is pretty well-established. Clinical trials have shown that the drug is as effective as lorazepam and alprazolam, and more effective than venlafaxine for GAD. Placebo-controlled trials have also shown that it is more effective than placebo for patients who have had only a partial response to SSRIs or SNRIs (for a recent review of these studies, see Reinhold & Rickels, 2015). Start at 100 mg QHS, and gradually titrate to 300 mg BID. Pregabalin's potential drawbacks in addition to its addictive properties include high rates of dizziness and sedation (20%–30% of patients), and an average weight gain of about 5 pounds after 4 weeks. There aren't any drug-drug interactions currently noted for pregabalin.

Gabapentin (Neurontin)

Gabapentin was originally used to prevent seizures as an anti-epilepsy drug. Its off-label uses include treatment for anxiety disorders as well as withdrawal from alcohol or benzodiazepines. (The drug was once also touted as a treatment for bipolar disorder, but well-designed trials discredited this use.) One small placebo-controlled trial found gabapentin (average dose 2,868 mg/day) superior to placebo for social phobia, but the response rates were low (32% for gabapentin, 14% for placebo) (Pande et al, 1999). For alcohol dependence, in one large double-blind trial, a rapid 4-day taper of gabapentin (from 1,200 mg/day to 800 mg/day) was more effective than a taper of lorazepam in terms of preventing relapse (Myrick et al, 2009). Common gabapentin side effects include dizziness and sedation, and there is increasing evidence that many patients abuse it for its sedative properties.

Quetiapine (Seroquel)

Quetiapine is hardly the first antipsychotic to be used or approved for anxiety. Stelazine (trifluoperazine) is approved for the short-term treatment of GAD, while Triavil (the combination of the antipsychotic perphenazine and the antidepressant amitriptyline) is approved for "depression and anxiety." In addition, many clinicians use low-dose chlorpromazine (Thorazine) off-label for anxiety. The advantage of quetiapine is that its efficacy evidence is more robust, with placebo-controlled trials of over 2,600 patients showing that the medication eases symptoms of GAD better than placebo, just as well as paroxetine, and better than escitalopram (for a review of these studies, see Gao et al, 2009). Lower doses of quetiapine XR, 50–150 mg QD, appear to be more effective than higher doses. Quetiapine has not won FDA approval for GAD, probably because its disadvantages literally outweigh its advantages (it's one of the worst antipsychotics in terms of weight gain and metabolic disturbances). Quetiapine, like gabapentin, has become a drug of abuse in some circles (Sansone & Sansone, 2010).

Natural medications

Don't forget to try some of the herbal medications. While they are not backed up by the same quantity or quality of randomized controlled trials we expect for conventional meds, many of them have a long history of safe and presumably effective use. As covered in the July/August 2013 issue of *The Carlat Psychiatry Report*, valerian root is often helpful for both sleep and anxiety. Its presumed mechanism of action is enhancing the action of GABA. Typical recommended doses include 450 mg of valerian extract at bedtime for sleep, and 200–300 mg in the morning for anxiety. Valerian is quite safe, though there have been very rare cases of mild liver enzyme elevations, which normalized after stopping the extract.

THE ART OF GENTLY REFUSING TO PRESCRIBE

Sometimes patients are insistent about requesting a medication we believe is inappropriate, and we have to refuse the request. The goal, of course, is to do so without completely alienating our patients. Here are some tricks of the trade.

• *Label controlled drugs as a second-line treatment.* You can frame the situation in terms of first-line vs. second-line treatment. Often I will use the concept of safety or health to reiterate that my treatment decisions are based on the patient's welfare. "Let's see if we can go with some healthier choices first." "At this point, let's try an alternative. Let's take the safe route and not risk relapsing." "We're going to attack the problem from a couple of different angles—one angle is to see if reducing the drinking helps."

• *Use the prescription as a carrot to stop substance use.* "I am willing to give you the benefit of the doubt, but I need to see something from you in return." That may mean an agreement to gradually taper down the use of the substance. And down the road, if drug screens have not shown success, you can say, "Because I'm not seeing a change in your behavior, that makes it hard for me to prescribe for you."

• *Refuse the prescription.* "I'm not going to prescribe you any benzodiazepines because I'm not comfortable with it until you've stopped using." You can soften the blow by offering a range of alternative medications, which gives your patient a sense of still having some control: "I won't be able to prescribe you Klonopin, but you can try Buspar, Neurontin, or Vistaril—which would you prefer?"

CASE CONCLUSION: *Because K's depression has not improved after a week, you begin a trial of citalopram. You also refer him to a psychologist to work on enhancing his coping skills for dealing with his depressed mood. It takes a while for K's depression to substantially remit, even with continued abstinence from alcohol, so in hindsight you surmise that he most likely had underlying depression in addition to alcohol use disorder.*

Self-Test Questions

1. A 30-year-old man presents for evaluation of worsening insomnia after stopping his cocaine use two months prior. He has a three-year history of intranasal cocaine use several times weekly, 4–6 beers per night, and occasional use of marijuana. Although he has stopped using cocaine, he continues to drink 2–3 beers several evenings per week to help him sleep. He denies problems with energy, motivation, or appetite, but he believes he is under surveillance by the FBI. He reports that the police on TV communicate with him through his TV set, and that the FBI is manipulating his thoughts with microwaves emitted from the cars across the street. Which of the following is the most likely diagnosis?
   a. Alcohol withdrawal syndrome
   b. Cocaine-induced depressive disorder
   c. Major depressive disorder
   d. Paranoid schizophrenia

2. A 42-year-old woman is evaluated one month after starting outpatient treatment for alcohol use disorder, and she has been abstinent since beginning treatment. She reports that she has lost interest in seeing friends and has been having feelings of guilt about her past since starting therapy. She cites difficulty sleeping at night, daytime fatigue, and loss of appetite that has led to recent unintentional weight loss. Which of the following is the most likely diagnosis for this patient?
   a. Alcohol protracted abstinence syndrome
   b. Major depressive disorder
   c. Dysthymia
   d. Adjustment disorder with depressed mood

3. A 25-year-old woman presents for evaluation because of a five-year history of alcohol and cocaine use disorder. Her longest period of abstinence was 30 days while in a residential addiction treatment program. She is currently in outpatient counseling, and she has reduced her use of alcohol and cocaine by half. However, she has begun feeling sad and hopeless, experiencing crying spells for no reason, and having no appetite. She reports that she sometimes wishes something bad would happen to her, and she has begun cutting herself with a knife when she gets too angry. She drinks daily to help calm her nerves, and lives with family

members who engage in heavy social drinking and do not participate in the patient's treatment. Which of the following is the most appropriate level of care for this patient?

a. Outpatient
b. Intensive outpatient
c. Long-term residential
d. Inpatient treatment in a dual diagnosis program

The answer key for these self-test questions is on page 233.

Note: If you purchased CME credit with this book, your CME post-test can be accessed when you are logged in at www.thecarlatreport.com/AddictionGuide. Please keep in mind that the question and answer order for that CME post-test are different than what you see in these self-test study questions.

CHAPTER 7

Alcohol

"That's the problem with drinking, I thought, as I
poured myself a drink. If something bad happens
you drink in an attempt to forget; if something good
happens you drink in order to celebrate; and if nothing
happens you drink to make something happen."
Charles Bukowski

TAKE HOME POINTS

- Ascertain your patient's pattern and amount of consumption in terms of standard drinks.
- Assess the chances that your patient will have significant withdrawal.
- Enhance your patient's motivation to decrease drinking.
- Choose outpatient or inpatient detox, depending on the severity of the problem.
- Choose among acamprosate, naltrexone, and disulfiram for support of ongoing recovery.

CASE VIGNETTE: *T is a 35-year-old man who is about to lose his wife due to his drinking. He began drinking beer in his college fraternity, and since then has not let a day go by without drinking. When I meet him for the first time, he tells me he has 2–3 mixed drinks each day, but each of T's drinks are sizable enough to be a couple drinks for someone else. He primarily drinks to help relieve stress and reduce his feelings of anxiety and depression. He thinks this helps get him through his day, but as we work together, he comes to realize that it is actually creating more problems.*

ESSENTIALS OF ALCOHOL

Take any source of sugar (grapes, wheat, potatoes, apples, and so on), leave it around to rot long enough, and you will surely create some alcohol. Typically, though, alcohol is produced through a more controlled process: washing the raw ingredients to minimize bacteria, adding yeast, keeping everything in a clean container, adding flavorants, and filtering out the undesirable parts of the plant (like stems and skins).

Alcohol has a pretty simple chemical formula: CH_3CH_2OH, which is an ethyl group linked to a hydroxyl group. The more precise term for it, therefore, is "ethanol," since alcohol technically refers to any organic compound attached to a hydroxyl group. Since it's more common, I'll use the term "alcohol" to refer to ethanol in this chapter.

Starches and yeast are abundant and have been for millennia, which explains why alcoholic beverages have been served since at least 7000 BC in Egypt. From a psychiatric point of view, alcohol became problematic as it grew more common, fueled in the 18th century in the United Kingdom, where gin consumption reached nearly 20 million gallons per year and alcoholism became widespread.

In 1920, the United States passed a law prohibiting the manufacture, sale, import, and export of intoxicating liquors. The illegal alcohol trade boomed, and by 1933, prohibition was lifted. Currently, 90% of U.S. men and 70% of U.S. women consume some form of alcohol, though most of them do not consume large amounts. In any given month, 23% of Americans binge drink, and 6% drink heavily.

Immediate effects

Alcohol acts rapidly because it is very lipid soluble. Cell membranes, with their lipid bilayers, offer almost no impediment to it. Alcohol's small size and lipid solubility make it pass the blood-brain barrier very quickly. Once in the brain, it stimulates some neurotransmitters and inhibits others. Alcohol's effects on the gamma-aminobutyric acid (GABA) receptor are what leads to its psychoactive effects. (For more detail on GABA, see Chapter 8 on sedatives.)

Though our knowledge of the neurobiology of alcohol is limited, we know plenty about its psychological effects. At low to moderate doses, alcohol creates relaxation and disinhibition. It is remarkably effective at reducing social anxiety, making it a staple at parties and earning it the nickname "the social lubricant." However, with greater consumption, alcohol's effects penetrate to progressively deeper parts of the brain. The effects start on the surface, at the frontal lobes, where it relaxes the executive functions. As the blood alcohol level rises, it quiets the reticular activating system, which is what keeps us awake and alert to our surroundings, so sedation ensues. Next, the cerebellum is affected, which impacts coordination and causes staggering. Ultimately, the brain stem is affected, which reduces the respiratory drive—at this point, we've reached the level of alcohol poisoning. Thankfully, alcohol poisoning (overdose) is fairly rare: Since alcohol is a liquid, a person must consume a large amount to produce the alcohol level necessary to overdose, and the body will generally expel the alcohol through vomiting before reaching that level.

Long-term effects

Long-term heavy alcohol use reduces an individual's lifespan by 10–15 years. See Table 7-1 for a rundown of the major organ systems that can be damaged by alcoholism.

As a psychiatrist, you are unlikely to be managing the complete treatment of all the various medical sequelae of alcohol use disorder. You will be more likely to address sequelae that affect the brain, such as alcohol-related dementia, but less likely to deal with liver disease or peripheral neuropathy. Your main job will be to ask medical screening questions, obtain appropriate labs, and refer patients to a primary care physician for follow-up if needed.

Some basic screening questions for alcohol-related syndromes include the following:

- Have you had yellow eyes? (jaundice)
- Have you had belly pain, especially on your right side, after drinking heavily? (acute alcoholic hepatitis)
- Have you had ulcers? Have you ever noticed dark stools or blood in your stool? (gastritis, gastrointestinal bleeding)
- Do you have a tendency to bruise or bleed easily? (low levels for clotting factors)
- Have you noticed numbness or tingling in your feet? (alcoholic neuropathy)
- Have you had memory or concentration problems? (alcohol-induced dementia)

TABLE 7-1. Some Common Medical Complications of Alcoholism

Liver disease. • Acute hepatitis. Liver cell destruction by alcohol; results in hepatic enzyme release from the liver; the typical symptom is right upper quadrant pain, and a typical sign is jaundice. • Cirrhosis. End stage of chronic liver disease; face may be red with "gin blossoms"— the dark, tortuous capillaries (also called spider angiomas) on the cheeks or other parts of the skin; abdominal enlargement due to build-up of ascitic fluid from liver failure.
Other GI issues. • Gastritis and peptic ulcer • Esophageal varices • Squamous cell cancer of the mouth and upper digestive tract
Peripheral neuropathy. Caused by neuron membrane damage by alcohol; presents in a stocking-glove distribution with numbness or tingling, first in the feet and later in the hands.

Alcoholic dementia and other brain disorders.
• Alcoholic dementia is a progressive cognitive decline accompanied by enlarged cerebral ventricles and sulci in the brain that occurs in heavy (5 or more standard drinks/day) drinkers and manifests as frontal lobe damage with difficulty planning and problem-solving, disinhibition, and reduced insight (Martin et al, 1986).
• Wernicke's encephalopathy (WE) is caused by thiamine (B1) deficiency and consists of the classic triad of ophthalmoplegia (eye muscle dysfunction), ataxia, and altered mental status.
  – It is a medical emergency requiring immediate treatment with parenteral thiamine (250 mg–500 mg daily for 3–5 days) to prevent development of Korsakoff's syndrome
  – Give thiamine before or concurrently with intravenous glucose, since giving glucose alone to a thiamine-deficient patient can precipitate Wernicke's encephalopathy due to thalamic neuronal damage (Thomson et al, 2002).
• Korsakoff's syndrome is a later manifestation of WE, and presents as memory loss that appears similar to dementia. It is the irreversible form of thiamine deficiency with chronic loss of working memory accompanied by confabulation (Sechi and Serra, 2007).

Labs you should consider ordering include a liver panel, which includes the transaminases, AST and ALT. Elevation of these enzymes is caused by leakage from damaged liver cells. Mild elevations are common and usually reversible with abstinence. Most concerning are elevations of four or more times the upper limit of normal (normal is defined by most labs as 40 or 50, so you would need to see transaminase levels of >200 to be concerned about acute hepatitis). Coagulation studies include PT, or INR. Elevation in these studies indicates more serious liver damage: In such a state, the liver is so damaged that it is not making coagulation factors, and a person will bruise easily due to "thin" blood that doesn't clot well.

CASE REVISITED: *Due to T's long history of alcohol consumption, I order a hepatic panel. It shows elevated transaminases of two to three times the upper limit of normal, but no coagulation abnormalities. We discuss these results, which were most likely due to alcohol consumption, either chronic liver damage or acute alcoholic hepatitis. The labs are a good opportunity for me to give T feedback about some consequences of his alcohol use.*

Withdrawal syndrome

Each patient will experience differing severity of alcohol withdrawal, ranging from nonexistent to life-threatening. Predicting the likelihood of withdrawal is more art than science. In general, patients who have consumed larger amounts for longer periods of time on a consistent basis will have more severe withdrawal. Binge drinkers will rarely have withdrawal symptoms other than a bad hangover.

Early symptoms occur within a few hours after the last drink—although it may take 24–48 hours for symptoms to manifest—and usually last 48–72 hours. They include insomnia, nervousness, tremor, and sweatiness. Early withdrawal symptoms may subside on their own, although repeated episodes of alcohol withdrawal increase the likelihood of progression to worse withdrawal, also known as late withdrawal or delirium tremens.

Heavier drinkers and those who have experienced repeated early withdrawal may experience delirium tremens, which starts after development of early withdrawal has continued to progress, usually 48–72 hours after the last drink. Also known as "the DTs," "the shakes," and "rum fits," symptoms of delirium tremens include worsening of the signs of early withdrawal, with serious altered mental status (hallucinations such as the famous "pink elephants") and severe autonomic dysregulation manifested by rapid fluctuations in vital signs. Development of delirium tremens carries a mortality of 5%, even when adequately treated. Because alcohol withdrawal can progress quickly and result in mortality, it is important to recognize and treat it early.

Seizures are an early sign of alcohol withdrawal syndrome and can complicate management. Patients who present with an alcohol withdrawal–related seizure or with delirium tremens should be treated as a medical emergency and referred to the nearest emergency department for adequate medical monitoring and aggressive pharmacologic management to prevent significant morbidity and mortality.

Alcoholic hallucinosis is a condition that can resemble alcohol withdrawal syndrome. It presents with auditory and/or visual hallucinations, but not the autonomic dysregulation of alcohol withdrawal syndrome. Alcoholic hallucinosis is not life-threatening and is a consequence of intoxication, but not withdrawal. It often resolves with resolution of intoxication over time, or with pharmacologic treatment to prevent alcohol withdrawal syndrome.

ASSESSMENT

In doing an alcohol assessment, your goals are:
1. Assess the amount and pattern of consumption
2. Assess whether the drinking is a problem (eg, whether the patient meets criteria for an alcohol use disorder)
3. Assess for the possibility of withdrawal

> ⬤ **CLINICAL PEARL: Alcohol Drug Screens— Are They Useful?**
>
> *When should you order an alcohol urine or blood screen, if at all?*
>
> *Urine alcohol screens are not useful because the detection window is short, less than 9 hours in most cases. A negative result won't tell you anything about your patient's drinking habits. A blood alcohol level is useful in an emergency room to evaluate a patient who seems to be acutely intoxicated, in order to see whether the behavior is due to alcohol, other drugs, or a medical condition. A breath alcohol level test, measured with a breathalyzer, is the simplest test for an office setting since it is comparable to a blood alcohol level. This is used mainly for patients who may be currently intoxicated when you need to decide whether they should drive and where they should go next.*

Initial questions

When asking about alcohol, I don't ask *whether* patients drink, but rather *how much* they drink. The vast majority of Americans drink at least occasionally, so it is not offensive to assume that a patient drinks.

Occasionally, patients will say they do not drink at all—approximately 15%–20% of people are "teetotalers." If someone says, "I don't drink," I want to find out why. Often, this choice is due to a previous bad experience with alcohol, although it can also be a family tradition or a religious edict.

Note, however, that sometimes the phrase "I don't drink" actually means the person doesn't drink very *often*. And even infrequent drinking can be a problem—for example, a patient may only drink once a year, but get into a car accident or some other kind of trouble during that time.

Patients will sometimes claim they are "social drinkers." If so, I follow up with questions like: "How often do you typically drink?" "When you drink, how much do you have?" and, "What's your favorite drink?"

You can use normalization by saying something like, "Lots of people drink—it's not unusual for people to have a six-pack a day." Patients may then feel more comfortable admitting to their actual usage: "Oh, no, I don't drink that much; I only have 4 beers each day."

The famous CAGE questionnaire can be used as a quick screening tool.

The CAGE Questionnaire

Cut down: "Have you felt you should cut down on your drinking?"

Annoyed: "Have people annoyed you by getting on your case about your drinking?"

Guilty: "Have you ever felt bad or guilty about your drinking?"

Eye-opener: "Have you ever needed to take a drink first thing in the morning to steady your nerves or get rid of a hangover?"

If a patient answers yes to 2 questions on the CAGE, or if someone age 65 or older answers yes to 1 question, these are triggers to probe further.

The best single screening question is, "How many times in the past year have you had X or more drinks in a day?" (where X = 5 for men and 4 for women). A positive response to this single-question screen was defined as 1 or more times (Smith et al, 2009).

Assessing consumption

Since alcohol use disorder is diagnosed based on whether alcohol is causing significant problems, a given amount of consumption doesn't necessarily signify a disorder. Nevertheless, we have some statistical benchmarks to help us interpret the significance of consumption. More importantly, quantifying consumption helps me predict how difficult it will eventually be for my patient to discontinue drinking—and how severe the withdrawal symptoms might be. By combining information about how much of a certain beverage a patient drinks, as well as how frequently, I will do a rough calculation of how many drinks the patient has per day or per week.

The Centers for Disease Control and Prevention defines excessive drinking as follows: For men, it is consumption of 15 or more "standard drinks" (SDs) in a week; for women, it is consumption of 8 or more SDs in a week. Excessive drinking correlates with a greater likelihood of having an alcohol problem (see the "Did You Know" chart for SD equivalents). (http://www.cdc.gov/alcohol/faqs.htm)

 DID YOU KNOW:
What Is a Standard Drink?

Beer
- 12 oz. can or bottle of beer up to 7% alcohol by volume = 1 standard drink (SD)
- 24 oz. beer, known as a "high boy," a deuce, or a double = 2 SDs
- A "pint" (usually comes in a large glass at a bar), 16 oz. = 1.3 SDs
- 36 oz. and 40 oz. containers = 3 to 3.5 SDs
- A case (24 beers) = 24 SDs

Wine
- 5 oz. of wine = 1 SD
- One bottle of wine (750 ml or 25 oz.) = 5 SDs
- A wine glass filled to the top (8 to 10 oz.) = about 2 SDs
- A champagne flute filled to the top (5 to 6 oz.) = 1 SD

Hard liquor
- 1 to 1.5 oz. = 1 SD
- A typical shot glass = 1 SD
- A typical mixed drink (2 to 3 oz. of alcohol) = about 2 SDs

CDC definitions for problem drinking
- Binging = 5 or more SDs on one occasion
- Excessive drinking = 15 or more SDs in a week (men), 8 or more SDs in a week (women)

In order to help assess withdrawal risk, I'll ask about the patient's recent pattern of drinking: "How much have you been drinking in the last 2 to 4 weeks? Has that pattern changed recently (up or down)?"

If someone drinks daily, I'll dig more deeply into questions pertaining to withdrawal symptoms: "What has been your longest period of abstinence? Have you been able to go for several days without a drink in the last 6 or 12 months?" "Have you been through alcohol withdrawal before?" If the patient doesn't know exactly what I mean, I'll use specific phrasing such as: "If you go without a drink for a day or two, do you get shaky or sweaty?"

Assessing consequences of drinking

Many of the DSM-5 criteria for alcohol use disorder have to do with negative consequences of drinking. Ask: "Have bad things happened to you as a result of drinking? Have you experienced any legal consequences, like a DUI? Have you had any relationship problems because of drinking?"

In my experience, patients don't always realize the negative consequences of their drinking. For example, a divorce may have been triggered by a patient's alcohol use, but unless the ex-spouse made this clear, the patient might not be aware of what caused the split. Other examples of consequences of drinking that may not be so obvious include:

• Not speaking to one's children for a prolonged period, perhaps because when the parent is drunk, the kids don't enjoy the interaction.
• Changing jobs frequently, possibly as a result of poor performance caused by frequent hangovers.

DSM-5 criteria

As you gain more experience evaluating alcohol-using patients, you will develop an interview approach that doesn't necessarily follow the DSM criteria in lockstep. Such interviews feel more natural and conversational. But initially, it's helpful to make sure you touch on each of the criteria, in part because you need to differentiate between mild use (2 criteria), moderate use (3–5), and severe use (more than 5).

I suggest keeping the criteria handy for reference. You can also use the mnemonic from Chapter 1: Tempted With Cocaine, Scotch, and Rum. This covers the major categories in DSM-5: Tolerance, Withdrawal, Control impairment, Social impairment, Risky behavior.

DSM-Focused Questions to Ask About Alcohol Use

Preliminary questions establishing amount of use:

- What is your favorite drink? What is your favorite brand of beer or whiskey?
- What time do you have your first drink? What time do you usually stop drinking for the day?

Questions about time spent obtaining alcohol (control impairment cluster):

- How often do you go to the liquor store?
- Do you hide your alcohol (beer/wine/whiskey) from your family?
- How long do you spend at the bar?
- Do you have cravings?
- Have you tried to cut down or quit drinking before?
- Do you often drink more than you really want to?

Questions about activities given up over time due to drinking (social impairment cluster):

- Are you spending less time with your family than before?
- Have you had to take time off from work because of drinking?
- Have you called in sick to work after drinking?
- Have you overslept for work or school after drinking?
- How much time do you spend socializing in settings that don't involve alcohol? Is this less time than before?
- Have you avoided going out because you prefer to stay home to drink?

Questions about use in hazardous (risky) situations:

- Have you ever driven after drinking? Have you ever had a DUI charge? Have you ever had a charge for being drunk in a public place (public intoxication)?
- Have you ever had to have a drink at work (or during the workday, such as on a lunch break)?
- Have you continued to use after a doctor told you about medical problems caused by drinking?

Questions about tolerance and withdrawal:

- How often do you have a hangover? How long does it take you to recover from a hangover?

- Have you had problems getting to sleep after drinking?
- Have you been through alcohol withdrawal before?
- Do you need to drink more than you previously did to get a buzz or drunk?
- What is the longest time you have been abstinent? How long ago was that?
- Who would support you if you decided to quit drinking now?

CASE REVISITED: *In talking with T, it is clear that he often craves alcohol and is drinking more than he had in the past, that his drinking is causing problems with his marriage, and that he has limited other activities (such as spending time with his children). He has unsuccessfully tried to cut back on his drinking, and he discloses that he'd once received a DUI charge. Since T meets 6 criteria from the DSM-5 list, I diagnose him with severe alcohol use disorder.*

TREATMENT

Assessing your patient's motivation

The first step in treatment is figuring out whether your patient is motivated to quit. The typical progression is to obtain data about the problematic aspects of your patient's use, and then to gently refer back to these issues in assessing insight and motivation. Here's a snippet from my interview with T to illustrate:

Doctor: It sounds like drinking has led to some problems for you.

Patient: A few.

Doctor: Do you think those problems are serious, or do you think you can continue drinking and do okay?

Patient: That's hard to say. I haven't lost my job or anything—it's not like I go to work drunk. I make a pretty good salary, and I provide for the family.

Doctor: That's true, but you did mention that your drinking has affected your relationships with your wife and your kids.

Patient: Yeah, that's been pretty rough lately.

Doctor: Given how much you value those relationships, do you think it's worth making another effort to look at your drinking?

Patient: I do want to try to cut down. I would really like to be able to have a drink socially, but I just can't seem to stop at one or two drinks.

Doctor: What do you think would tell you that it's time to quit drinking altogether?

Patient: If my wife left me. And I think she's pretty close to that.

> ⭕ **CLINICAL PEARL: Dealing With an Intoxicated Patient**
>
> *How would you deal with an intoxicated patient in your office? First, try to gently isolate the patient from others in the waiting area, especially if the patient is disruptive. Assess whether the patient poses a threat. For example, if the patient is accompanied by a minor, you should call the police or the local Child Protective Services. The impaired patient should not be allowed to drive. This may involve having a family member or friend pick up the patient from the office, calling a taxi, or arranging for suitable public transportation. Of note, if a patient is intoxicated in the office, then by definition that patient has unhealthy alcohol use, so this can be addressed clinically and used to motivate the patient to consider a change to healthier behavior (Weaver, 2013).*

Planning a treatment strategy

Sometimes a patient's goal is to return to controlled drinking, as T hints in the above interview. While it's good to be flexible and to meet your patients where they are, in practice controlled drinking isn't usually possible for those with severe drinking problems, so initially I encourage at least a temporary trial of abstinence.

Some patients may be able to gradually cut down their drinking without any particular detox protocol. It may be reasonable to say, "Try cutting down on your own and start by going from 6 beers a day to 5 beers a day." In some cases, patients will surprise you and exceed your expectations—maybe even cutting down to 4 or 3 beers a day. But if they are unable to accomplish their goal, you can use that as a rationale for recommending more support, such as Alcoholics Anonymous meetings or individual or group therapy.

Detox: Outpatient vs. inpatient

Detox is medically supervised withdrawal, and can be done either as an outpatient or inpatient. How do you decide which is appropriate?

Inpatient detox is best for patients with the following characteristics:

- Significant consistent alcohol use daily for months. Such patients are at higher risk for severe withdrawal symptoms.
- History of seizures, whether from alcohol withdrawal or some other cause.
- Medical comorbidities: heart disease, liver disease, diabetes, other unstable medical problems, or taking multiple medications.
- Psychiatric comorbidities: severe anxiety, psychotic disorder, potential for suicidal ideation, or taking multiple medications.
- Unstable home environment: homelessness, lack of supportive friends or family members.
- Unreliability: unable to call the office, lack of transportation, unable to follow all instructions for an outpatient taper.

Conversely, an outpatient taper is usually fine for medically healthy patients who have no history of seizures, are reliable, and have fairly good psychosocial supports.

Inpatient and outpatient detox are both based on gradually tapering the doses of sedative medications. But whereas outpatient detox uses a fixed-dose protocol (more on this later), inpatient units generally use symptom-triggered protocols, meaning that they will choose dosages of medications based on the severity of withdrawal symptoms. The assessment tool most often used is the CIWA-Ar (Clinical Institute Withdrawal Assessment for Alcohol, revised), sometimes just called the CIWA (see Appendix), which requires trained staff to rate the severity of 10 specific withdrawal symptoms:

- Nausea and vomiting
- Tremor
- Sweats
- Anxiety
- Agitation
- Tactile disturbances
- Auditory disturbances
- Visual disturbances

- Headache
- Orientation and clouded sensorium

Each item is rated from 0 (not present) to 7 (most severe), with the exception of the sensorium item, which is rated from 0 to 4. The highest possible score is 67. Based on the score, the patient is given a prespecified sedative dose and frequency.

Because of the intensity of medical supervision, inpatient detox can be done quickly, taking 3–5 days in most cases, as opposed to the 5–10 days for outpatient detox.

Outpatient detox

Outpatient detox uses a fixed-dose protocol—you tell your patient at the beginning what the dose and frequency will be. Patients are allowed to take extra doses as needed if they have withdrawal symptoms.

The first decision is which cross-dependent medication to substitute for the alcohol. There are several effective options, but they are all fairly long-acting sedatives. It is less important which medication you use and more important that you are comfortable using it.

The most common medications used for detox are diazepam (Valium), chlordiazepoxide (Librium), and to a lesser extent, clonazepam (Klonopin). They are popular because they are long-acting, resulting in serum levels staying fairly high between doses and producing a smoother withdrawal. Lorazepam (Ativan) and oxazepam (Serax) are also sometimes used. Although both of them are short-acting, they have the advantage of requiring minimal liver metabolism, which makes them good choices for patients with liver disease.

My go-to detox sedative is actually none of the benzodiazepines, but phenobarbital, a barbiturate. Phenobarbital is an ideal detox medication for a number of reasons:

1. Phenobarbital is less addictive than the benzodiazepines, because it has a more gradual onset, generally an hour or more (as phenobarbital takes longer to cross the blood-brain barrier than benzos). It thus causes less euphoria than Valium or Librium, making it less likely to be abused. In addition, phenobarbital is generally less prescribed, which means less of it is available for diversion—this makes it less likely that a patient detoxed on this drug will be able to obtain it for later misuse.

2. Phenobarbital is safer in patients with liver damage. Both Valium and Librium are dependent on the liver for metabolism, whereas about 30% of phenobarbital is excreted unchanged. This means that Valium and Librium accumulate more than phenobarbital in such patients.

3. Phenobarbital has the longest half-life of any detox sedative—about 100 hours on average. This allows for less frequent dosing, and also means that many patients can simply stop phenobarbital without tapering, since its gradual metabolism leads to a natural metabolic tapering.

4. Dosing of phenobarbital is easier because it produces no active metabolites. Both Valium and Librium are converted by the liver into active metabolites, which complicates the dosing, especially in patients with any amount of liver impairment. Impaired liver function delays the clinical effect, and can lead to the erroneous conclusion that detoxing patients need more of the drug.

Some physicians are skeptical of using phenobarbital because of barbiturates' reputation for abuse and overdose. This reputation is based on barbiturates such as secobarbital (Seconal), which is highly addictive because it has a short half-life. Phenobarbital, meanwhile, has the longest half-life of any barbiturate.

Procedure for outpatient detox

Whether you favor a benzodiazepine or phenobarbital for detox, the procedure is similar for all sedatives. Start by prescribing a larger "loading dose" regimen initially. The size of the initial "loading" doses will vary depending on how much tolerance your patient has developed.

Start by prescribing the loading dose regimen with medication taken every 6 hours. Using phenobarbital as an example, a typical loading regimen is 30 mg (two 15 mg pills) Q 6 hours. I will generally write an initial prescription for thirty 15 mg pills with no refills, with the expectation that I will see the patient back in the office the next day. In determining the initial dose needed, it is better to err on the side of giving more rather than not enough. Why? Because if patients take too much, they will simply fall asleep; but if they do not have enough, they are at risk for a withdrawal seizure.

With the first dose or two, patients may not notice any effect from the medication, aside from having no withdrawal symptoms (they may notice a slight euphoric effect on benzodiazepines). Tell patients that if they feel shaky or sweaty after the first couple of doses, it's okay to take an extra 15 mg tab between doses. When I see them the next day, I'll find out how many extra doses they took and adjust the standing dose accordingly. My goal is to make sure withdrawal symptoms are suppressed while avoiding oversedation.

Maintain the standing dose for a few days, then begin a gradual taper. Here's how to do it. Let's assume that you started your patient on phenobarbital 2 days ago, and you've settled on a standing dose of two 15 mg tabs 4 times a day—typically at 6 am, 12 pm, 6 pm, and 12 am. One option is to direct your patient to simply decrease by a pill a day, letting them decide which dose to lower first. But I have had more success by being quite specific. Patients generally do better when they start by decreasing the daytime doses, reserving the nighttime dose taper for last. See Table 7-2 below for my usual recommendations.

TABLE 7-2. Outpatient Alcohol Detox Regimen With Phenobarbital

	Day 1	Day 2	Day 3	Day 4	Day 5	Day 6	Day 7	Day 8	Day 9	Day 10
6 am	15, 15	15, 15	15, 15	15, 15	15	15	15 three times daily	15 twice daily	15 once daily	15 once every few days until discontinue
12 pm	15, 15	15, 15	15	15	15	15				
6 pm	15, 15	15, 15	15, 15	15	15	15				
12 am	15, 15	15, 15	15, 15	15, 15	15, 15	15				

Notes: "15" refers to 15 mg phenobarbital. "Day 1" etc are illustrative and may need adjusting in patients who cannot tolerate this rapid a taper rate.

Recommended loading doses of other sedatives:
- Valium, 20 mg Q 6 hours
- Librium, 50 mg Q 6 hours
- Klonopin, 0.5 mg–1 mg Q 6 hours

The 10-day taper is fairly conservative, and when you use long-acting sedatives for the taper, you can speed up the process. Another approach is a very rapid "load and go" method, in which you give two days of an initial larger "loading dose" and then stop completely. Be careful, though—this is primarily an option with phenobarbital, since it is metabolized very gradually, allowing for a biological self-taper.

Using non-sedatives for detox

There are several non-sedatives that are sometimes used for detox, either as a replacement for sedatives or as an adjunct. Anticonvulsants are the most popular, primarily gabapentin (Neurontin) and carbamazepine (Tegretol). The advantage of using these types of medications is that they are not as addictive as sedatives (though gabapentin is increasingly becoming a drug of abuse in some settings). The disadvantage is that there is less evidence on the effectiveness of these agents and far less clinical experience.

Comfort medications

Some clinicians prescribe "comfort meds" to make detox easier. In my experience, if you are using sufficient doses of sedatives, patients will not need such meds. Nonetheless, here are some of the typical symptoms and meds used:
- Nausea: metoclopramide 10 mg; ondansetron 4 mg
- Insomnia: trazodone 50 mg; diphenhydramine 50 mg
- Anxiety: clonidine

CASE REVISITED: *I start T on phenobarbital and give him a prescription to take two 15 mg tablets at a time every 6 hours. The next day, I see him and determine that he is not having any signs of alcohol withdrawal (no tremor, no sweating, minimal anxiety, and no hallucinations; his vital signs, which my clinic staff took in the office, are well within the normal range). He says that he had awakened in the middle of the night and taken an extra phenobarbital tablet, which helped him go back to sleep. I have him continue taking phenobarbital at the prescribed dose of 2 tablets every 6 hours for another 48 hours. On the third day after starting the prescription, T sees me in the office again and reports no withdrawal symptoms—he also claims he's sleeping better than he had in years. I have him gradually reduce his total daily dose of phenobarbital by 1 tablet every 2 days over the next 2 weeks, which he tolerates without difficulty.*

Medication-assisted treatment for alcoholism

In this section, I'll go through the three main medications that are used to treat underlying alcohol use disorder: naltrexone, acamprosate, and disulfiram.

In my experience, most patients can benefit from one of these medications. Before starting any of them, I tell patients that the meds should not be used alone, but as an adjunct to some type of behavioral treatment. In this way, they serve a dual purpose: They are inherently effective, but they also keep patients engaged in a more comprehensive treatment program.

When I'm introducing pharmacotherapy, I'll start by asking, "Have you heard about some of the treatment options out there?" "Is there a medication you've heard about that you're interested in trying?" Some patients may have heard or read about these medications and have preferences—perhaps they've tried or been offered them before. For example, I had a patient who had been offered Vivitrol at a detox facility and turned it down, but was ready to give it a try when he saw me because of his lack of success quitting without it.

I'll also ask, "Are you aware that there are medications that are proven to be helpful?" Sometimes, I will briefly describe some of the research on medications for alcoholism. For example, the COMBINE trial randomized patients to naltrexone and acamprosate; naltrexone was somewhat more effective, and combining the two medications was not significantly more effective than either one alone.

Naltrexone oral (ReVia)

🔍 **NALTREXONE ORAL (REVIA)—AT A GLANCE**	
Indication	Alcohol dependence
Dosages available	50 mg
Target dose	Start and maintain 50 mg/day
Comments	No significant interactions other than avoiding use with opiates

Naltrexone is a long-acting version of the opioid blocker naloxone. Some of the euphoriant effects of alcohol are mediated through endogenous opioids, and naltrexone therefore blocks some of what makes drinking fun. Patients will take that first drink, and it won't give them a significant buzz; this helps to give them time to think about what they are doing and to decrease consumption. It also helps to reduce cravings for alcohol. Here's how I often describe naltrexone's effects: "It doesn't make you feel bad if you drink, it just doesn't let drinking make you feel good."

The oral version of naltrexone is a 50 mg pill that patients take once a day. Taking it at the same time every day is a good idea to prevent forgetting a dose, and ideally, someone should watch the patient take it to ensure accountability. The only common side effect is nausea, which goes away after a few days. Taking it with food helps diminish the nausea—I tell patients to start eating their meal, take the pill halfway through, then finish the meal.

While there's a small incidence of elevated liver enzymes as a side effect, there's no requirement to either get baseline enzymes or to monitor those labs. In practice, I will often check baseline LFTs initially (especially in patients with a history of liver problems), but in healthy patients with good medical care I will not always order those labs. Liver disease per se is not a contraindication to taking naltrexone. I will order follow-up LFTs in such patients only if there's a clinical prompt—ie, if there are complaints suggestive of liver damage. In my many years of experience prescribing this medication, I've never come across any liver problems caused by naltrexone. However, you can't go wrong by checking a liver panel, so I have a low threshold to do so, including if the patient has any concerns.

Some clinicians advise patients to take naltrexone as needed before situations, such as parties, where they will be tempted by alcohol. While this approach might be helpful for some patients, I'm personally not a big fan of it, because there's not much evidence that it supports recovery, and I'm concerned that it implicitly gives patients "permission" to put themselves in situations where there's a lot of alcohol. Nonetheless, if someone has been stable in recovery for a while, the as-needed approach may make more sense.

Naltrexone injectable (Vivitrol)

🔍 NALTREXONE INJECTABLE (VIVITROL)—AT A GLANCE	
Indication	Alcohol dependence
Dosages available	380 mg
Target dose	380 mg IM (gluteal) Q 4 weeks
Comments	No significant interactions other than avoiding use with opiates

The IM version comes in a standard 380 mg vial and is given once every 4 weeks. The main advantage of the shot is that it ensures a good serum level of the medication over that time frame. In addition, the shot entails a lower total dose of medication, if you're concerned about liver damage.

To order the medication, go to the manufacturer's website, www.vivitrol. com, which will guide you through the process. Generally, the vials will be delivered to your office about a week after the prescription. This depends on the patient's health care insurance coverage (including Medicaid), so patients may need to pick up the Vivitrol at a pharmacy and bring it to your office. It comes in two vials that must be refrigerated, one liquid, the other powder. Let it warm up to room temperature, which takes 45 minutes or so. When your patient is ready, dissolve the powder into the liquid, mix it, and draw it up in a syringe. Have the patient lay down and expose the upper outer quadrant of the buttock. Giving the shot resembles the wrist action involved in throwing a dart. The needle goes in quickly and smoothly, then pull back on the syringe plunger to check for blood return to make sure you are in the muscle and not a blood vessel. You take a few seconds to inject the medication, pull out the needle quickly, and massage the medication into the muscle. It's not a particularly painful injection, and although there have been reports of injection site problems, I've never seen them. I see patients within a week after the first shot, just to make sure they're tolerating it and have not had an injection site reaction; after that, they come back every 4 weeks for the injection.

The major thing to tell patients is that if they have an injury requiring opioid analgesics, they will need a higher opioid dose than usual to overcome the opioid receptor blockade. The manufacturer provides a wrist band, wallet card, or necklace tag ("dog tag") for patients to wear so treating physicians know they are taking Vivitrol.

Regardless of which formulation patients take, they should give it about a 6-month trial with an option to extend another 3–6 months.

Acamprosate (Campral)

ACAMPROSATE (CAMPRAL)—AT A GLANCE	
Indication	Alcohol dependence
Dosages available	333 mg (delayed-release tablets)
Target dose	666 TID mg/day
Comments	Give 333 mg TID in patients with renal impairment

Acamprosate's mechanism of action is not well-defined, but it seems to work on the glutamate neurotransmitter system. It is effective at decreasing cravings for alcohol. The most common thing I hear from patients taking it is, "I just don't think much about drinking anymore." Interestingly, if patients take acamprosate for 12 months, then stop it, the effect continues for another 12 months, implying that the medication causes some long-term changes in the brain.

In general, I find acamprosate more useful than naltrexone. There are no side effects aside from loose stools when patients start taking it, no drug interactions, no liver issues, and no issues with interfering with the effectiveness of analgesics—however, it is necessary to lower the dose if a patient has significant kidney problems. The disadvantage to acamprosate, though, is the larger pill burden. Patients must take 2 of the 333 mg pills three times a day, and they are large pills. I tell patients, "It's three times a day: breakfast, lunch, and dinner." On the positive side, some patients say it reminds them throughout the day that they are working on something to stop drinking.

As an aside, some patients find it amusing that the usual number of mg per dose of acamprosate is 666, which some people associate with Satan and all things immoral. It's not a reason to avoid prescribing it!

Disulfiram (Antabuse)

🔍 DISULFIRAM (ANTABUSE)—AT A GLANCE	
Indication	Alcohol dependence
Dosages available	250 mg, 500 mg tablets
Target dose	125 mg QPM–500 mg QPM
Comments	Must be abstinent from alcohol for at least 12 hours to start; maintenance therapy may be required for months or even years

Antabuse (disulfiram) interferes with the metabolism of alcohol and leads to an accumulation of acetaldehyde, which is similar to formaldehyde (embalming fluid). It is classified as an aversive agent; it conditions people not to drink because drinking becomes unpleasant. If someone does drink on Antabuse, the reaction feels a lot like having a heart attack, with chest tightness, palpitations, shortness of breath, nausea, and a bad headache.

Antabuse is prescribed as a 500 mg tablet once a day. It's best in a monitored setting, where the patient can be observed taking it every day. After stopping the medication, it takes several days to wear off. The medication is contraindicated for people with significant heart disease, and must be given at a lower dose (250 mg) in people with liver disease. It can also worsen psychotic features.

You should warn patients that many over-the-counter medicines contain alcohol and can cause a reaction if they are taking Antabuse, such as Vicks Formula 44 cough syrup (the "44" is the proof of the alcohol in it). Anything that says "elixir" should be avoided, because that term means the medicine is dissolved in alcohol. Even things like rum cake can cause a reaction.

I tend not to use Antabuse as much as other meds. The last patient I prescribed it for had continued drinking despite being on Vivitrol for over a year and decided he needed something more definitive. He responded to Antabuse well. He had one reaction to it after a couple of months, when he went to a golf tournament and decided to have a couple of drinks. Nothing terrible happened—he felt very bad and went straight home.

CASE CONCLUSION: *After he completes his phenobarbital detox, I see T again to discuss long-term options for treatment of his alcohol use disorder. He is going to Alcoholics Anonymous and has a therapist, and he asks me what medications might help him with his sobriety. We talk about the pros and cons of disulfiram, naltrexone, and acamprosate. He is not interested in disulfiram because he does not want to risk having a serious reaction if he does have a drink, and he is not interested in Vivitrol because he doesn't want to have shots. Since he is still struggling with alcohol cravings, I recommend acamprosate. T is somewhat reluctant to consider a medication that must be taken three times a day, but he likes the idea that he would only have to take it for 12 months and that the effects would continue afterward. I explain that most patients take acamprosate with breakfast, lunch, and dinner so that it is easier to remember, and he agrees to try it. He does not have any problems with side effects, and within a week he notices his cravings to drink are almost completely gone. Over the next couple of years, T successfully abstains from alcohol and is able to spend more time with his daughters—which he finds much more enjoyable than drinking.*

Self-Test Questions

1. A 45-year-old man with alcohol use disorder is considering starting acamprosate. He takes lisinopril for high blood pressure, and routine blood work by his primary care physician was normal except for mild elevation in liver transaminases. The patient asks what precautions he should take while on acamprosate. Which of the following is the most important information to give him?
   a. The effectiveness of opioid analgesics may be reduced
   b. Ingestion of alcohol may cause flushing and chest tightness
   c. Taking lisinopril may reduce the effectiveness of acamprosate
   d. There are no significant drug interactions

2. You are seeing a 35-year-old woman for a new patient evaluation. She requests a prescription for alprazolam (Xanax) "for her nerves." When you ask what else she has done to help with her nerves, she tells you she has several mixed drinks after work and before going to bed. You decide to screen for an alcohol use disorder by asking her the CAGE questionnaire. Which of the following questions do you ask this patient?
   a. Have you ever felt you've lost control of your drug use?
   b. Have you ever accepted money or drugs for sex to pay for your use?
   c. Have you ever felt guilty about your drug use?
   d. Have you ever felt enraged by other people criticizing your drug use?

3. A 48-year-old man with a history of alcoholic hepatitis and alcohol use disorder sees you for a follow-up evaluation because of alcohol craving. He had been drinking up to one liter of vodka daily. Six days ago, the patient was discharged from a two-week hospitalization for acute alcohol-induced pancreatitis that was complicated by alcohol withdrawal and aspiration pneumonia. He has been abstinent since hospital discharge, but asks for help with his alcohol cravings. Which of the following is the most appropriate pharmacotherapy to help prevent this patient from relapsing?
   a. Disulfiram
   b. Fluoxetine
   c. Naltrexone
   d. Topiramate

The answer key for these self-test questions is on page 233.

Note: If you purchased CME credit with this book, your CME post-test can be accessed when you are logged in at www.thecarlatreport.com/AddictionGuide. Please keep in mind that the question and answer order for that CME post-test are different than what you see in these self-test study questions.

CHAPTER 8

Sedatives

"But one led to two, two led to four, four led to eight, until at
the end it was about 85 a day—the doctors could not believe
I was taking that much. And that was just the Valium—
I'm not talking about the other pills I went through."

Corey Haim, actor

TAKE HOME POINTS

- The most commonly abused sedatives are alprazolam, diazepam, chlordiazepoxide, and zolpidem.
- The usual detox regimen for sedatives uses phenobarbital.
- There is no medication treatment for sedative use disorder; neither naltrexone nor acamprosate is effective.

CASE VIGNETTE: *H is a 23-year-old single male referred to me by his family because of their concerns about his drug use. He lives with his mother and works as a cook in his uncle's restaurant. He tells me that as a teenager he had used alcohol and marijuana, but not excessively, aside from occasional binges with friends. But things changed at about age 17, when a friend gave him alprazolam (Xanax) to try. He enjoyed how it made him feel, so he started using it daily, and would also use zolpidem (Ambien). The alprazolam took the place of most of his alcohol use. As he developed tolerance to the alprazolam, he began using it multiple times a day, generally using 10 mg per day. Eventually H switched from oral use to intranasal snorting of the tablets, because it provided a more rapid onset of euphoria.*

ESSENTIALS OF SEDATIVES

The sedative-hypnotics include the benzodiazepines, the Z-drugs (so named because they all have the letter Z in the generic name), and the barbiturates. Ethanol, covered in Chapter 7, is also often classified as a sedative—specifically a liquid, as opposed to the solid sedatives we'll cover in this chapter.

Immediate effects

All sedatives, solid or liquid, initially produce a sense of euphoria, well-being, and disinhibition. They are most often prescribed to reduce anxiety and sleeplessness.

At high doses, sedatives can cause anterograde amnesia, which means the user stops recording memories despite being awake and alert, so that there is no memory of events during the time of the sedative effect. With heavy alcohol use, this is known as a "blackout," which is not the same thing as "passing out" (oversedation). Patients who abuse sedatives may not realize they have had a blackout until someone "reminds" them of things they said or did during an amnesic period. I tell patients that this is like having a "Swiss cheese memory" with holes in it, except that the memory gaps aren't always obvious because "you don't remember what you don't remember" while using. As the dosage increases, these drugs cause increasing sedation and central nervous system depression, and can eventually lead to an overdose syndrome of profound sedation, respiratory depression, and death.

Pharmacologically, sedatives cause these effects presumably by affecting the gamma-aminobutyric acid (GABA) receptor system. GABA is the major inhibitor neurotransmitter in the brain, and it serves as a natural counterbalance to the many excitatory neurotransmitters, such as glutamate. When GABA latches onto its receptors, it causes an ion channel to open up, which in turn allows negative chloride ions to enter the neuron. This hyperpolarizes the neuron, which is the opposite of the more famous depolarization process that causes neurons to fire. Hyperpolarization inhibits action potentials and keeps neurons quiescent.

Like all neurotransmitter systems, GABA receptors are complicated. There are two classes (GABA A and GABA B), each with multiple subunits. Our current understanding is that benzodiazepines work by altering the shape of the receptor so that GABA can inhibit neurons more efficiently.

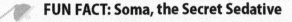

FUN FACT: Soma, the Secret Sedative

Carisoprodol (Soma) is prescribed as a muscle relaxant for the treatment of acute musculoskeletal pain. Many physicians are unaware that the liver metabolizes it into meprobamate, which used to be a very popular sedative sold as Miltown or Equanil. Since carisoprodol is not an obvious sedative medication, it is often sought by patients trying to scam their doctors and eventually ends up on the black market. Cyclobenzaprine (Flexeril) and baclofen (Lioresal) are also muscle relaxants, but they don't have metabolites with sedative properties, so they are not particularly popular among drug abusers.

The Z-drugs do something similar, but are more selective than benzos because they are limited to one particular subunit that causes sleepiness—whereas benzos also attach to subunits that soothe anxiety, relax muscles, and prevent seizures. Barbiturates are the hammers of sedatives, because they have a double-whammy effect of enhancing GABA's efficiency as well as *directly* activating the chloride channel.

All sedatives are potentially addictive, though some appear to be more "liked" by substance users than others. The likability of sedatives is often correlated with how quickly they start working. For example, alprazolam has a very rapid onset of action and is probably the most popular sedative on the black market. When the Z-drugs were first introduced, they were marketed as having little if any abuse potential, but over time it has become clear that they are abusable, and that they cause both tolerance and withdrawal symptoms.

Barbiturates are still around, but they are rarely used in psychiatry because the short-acting version, secobarbital (Seconal), turned out to be highly addictive and often lethal in overdose. These days, barbiturates are most commonly prescribed for seizures, headaches (the migraine pill Fioricet contains butalbital, which is a short-acting barbiturate, in addition to acetaminophen and caffeine), anesthesia, and alcohol withdrawal.

Long-term effects

Multiple studies have shown an association between long-term use of benzodiazepines and development of dementia when compared to those who have not used benzodiazepines (Zhong et al, 2015). Benzodiazepine use can as much as double the risk for dementia (Billioti de Gage et al, 2015). The mechanism for this is not yet known, nor is it completely clear that this is a cause-effect relationship, rather than just a correlation. Nonetheless, the research is concerning, and sharing the information with patients may help motivate them to stop chronic benzodiazepine use.

ASSESSMENT

Diagnosing sedative use disorder is straightforward for patients who are using large amounts and who are forthcoming about their use. The case vignette at the beginning of this chapter is typical for such patients. H describes his history of Xanax use in detail. In terms of formally diagnosing the DSM disorder and assigning a level of severity, I usually obtain this information in the context of asking general questions about the patient's pattern of use.

CASE REVISITED: *As I continue talking to H, I learn aspects of his history relevant to his DSM diagnosis, without asking him questions pegged to each of the criteria. Below, I've listed some elements of his history. Your job is to figure out which DSM criteria are relevant to each element (the answers follow the first list).*

---

1. He has tried to cut down his Xanax use more than once, but he became so unpleasantly sweaty and tremulous that he abandoned the efforts.
2. His use has increased to snorting about 10 mg per day.
3. He is worried about nodding off around the hot stove in the restaurant, yet he still uses on work days.
4. His use occasionally causes him to miss work days.
5. Both his mother and uncle are concerned about his job performance and behavior, resulting in frequent arguments with both of them.
6. He has been stopped for driving while intoxicated and is awaiting a court date.
7. He has cravings for Xanax (I actually asked him specifically about this: "Do you have cravings to use when you don't have it available?")

Ascertaining craving can be tricky, because patients may not understand what the term means and may inaccurately answer "no" when asked about it. If you suspect that craving might be present, it's worth explaining what it is in more detail. You can say something like, "Craving means the experience of really wanting to use a substance. That desire can be triggered by an emotion, like feeling anxious and craving Xanax. Or it can be triggered by a situation that reminds you of using the drug, like being in your bathroom if that is where you normally ingest it. Do you tend to have these craving experiences?"

Here are the DSM-5 criteria for sedative use disorder (see Chapter 1 for a mnemonic to help remember these criteria). Based on his history, how many criteria does H meet?

1. **Tolerance.** Yes, he has increased his use to continue to feel the high.
2. **Withdrawal syndrome.** Yes, he has felt sweaty and shaky.
3. **Cravings.** Yes, I asked about this specifically.
4. **Using more than planned.** Yes, anyone who is snorting Xanax 5 times a day is using more than planned!
5. **Unable to quit despite attempts.** Yes, he told me he had unsuccessfully tried to quit.
6. **Much time spent obtaining or recovering from substance.** No information.
7. **Important social, occupational, or recreational activities given up or reduced because of substance use.** Unclear.
8. **Failure to fulfill major role obligations at work, school, or home.** Yes, he has missed work occasionally.
9. **Persistent social and interpersonal problems caused by substance.** Probably, since his use has led to arguments with his mother and uncle.
10. **Substance use continued despite the patient's knowledge of significant physical or psychological problems caused by its use.** Unclear.
11. **Recurrent substance use in physically hazardous situations.** Yes, he has used while driving (hence the court date) and while cooking over a hot stove.

Counting them up, H fulfills 8 of the 11 criteria, placing him in the severe sedative use disorder category.

TREATMENT

In treating sedative addiction, there are two phases to consider: withdrawal/detox and relapse prevention. Before starting treatment for a patient such as H, I use the "good things and less-good things" motivational interviewing technique in order to help him see the advantages of quitting, as illustrated here:

Doctor: What do you like about your use of Xanax?

H: I like being high, it lifts me up when I'm stressed out, and also my friends are doing it and I like doing it with them.

Doctor: What are some less-good aspects of Xanax?

H: It's a bummer when my mom gets on my case about being asleep when I'm supposed to be doing something for her. And I don't like it when my uncle yells at me when I'm late for work. I also hate the withdrawals when I can't get it.

Sedative detox

The withdrawal syndrome due to sedatives is similar to alcohol withdrawal syndrome. If you think of alcohol as a liquid sedative, its time course and manifestations are similar to a short-acting sedative. Longer-acting sedatives such as diazepam or chlordiazepoxide may take longer to develop clear symptoms of withdrawal (3–6 days instead of 1–2 days after the last use), but the symptoms will be similar to alcohol withdrawal with elevations in vital signs, diaphoresis, and mild alteration of mental status initially, followed by worsening delirium and autonomic dysregulation as withdrawal progresses. Sedative withdrawal can be fatal, so rapid recognition and prevention or treatment are essential.

First you must determine whether the patient is a candidate for outpatient detox, and if so, choose a long-acting sedative to use for the taper. Although benzodiazepines are often used for alcohol withdrawal, they are not great choices for benzodiazepine withdrawal because of the risk of fueling the addiction. The most common choice is phenobarbital. Choosing the right loading dose requires knowing the equivalent sedative doses (see Table 8-1, "Characteristics of Commonly Used Sedatives," later in the chapter).

CASE REVISITED: *After further discussion, H elects to proceed with an outpatient detox. It is clear that he is at risk for withdrawal. Since he is young and healthy and has a supportive living situation, I use an outpatient phenobarbital load and taper. Because H is taking 10 mg of Xanax per day, and 1 mg of Xanax is roughly equivalent to 15 mg* *of phenobarbital, the phenobarbital equivalent would be 150 mg in a 24-hour period. However, since H also occasionally uses alcohol and Ambien, I increase his loading dose to 180 mg, or 60 mg every 8 hours.*

A loading dose regimen allows you to fairly rapidly (over 8–12 hours) achieve a medication dose level that matches the patient's level of tolerance in order to completely suppress sedative withdrawal symptoms. This works best with long-acting sedatives because they work more slowly in terms of initial onset of effect; thus, larger initial doses do not cause an overdose, but "stack up" on one another. Of course, you have to be careful not to give doses that are too high, because that could result in excess accumulation in the blood. The key is to carefully assess patients' level of tolerance, which is reflected by the dosage of illicit sedatives they are currently taking. As long as you match the loading dose of the detox medication with their current "street" dosing, it is extremely unlikely that you will cause an overdose.

After you have given the loading dose, you have two options: load and taper, or load and go. Load and taper is the more common method (see Chapter 7, Table 7-2: "Outpatient Alcohol Detox Regimen With Phenobarbital"). Load and go means giving the loading dose and then stopping all meds, allowing the medication to gradually metabolize out of the system (sometimes known as "self-tapering"). This method only works with sedatives with very long half-lives, such as phenobarbital and clonazepam.

Regardless of the method you use, when starting an outpatient detox, it is crucial that you give patients clear instructions and that the patient is capable of strictly complying with them. Taking too little of the detox medication can lead to worsening of sedative withdrawal syndrome, which can be fatal. Taking too much of the detox medication or combining it with other sedatives (including the one that was being abused) can result in an overdose, which can also be fatal. I inform my patient about this prior to starting the detox. If I don't trust the patient to be compliant with taking the medication as instructed or to at least call me if there are problems, then it is not safe and I will recommend an inpatient detox. I also tell patients that taking the detox medication is an all-or-nothing choice: If they take it, they must not take any other sedative for any reason. I tell them that if they change their mind and decide to go back to using the sedative that they were abusing, then they must stop the taper and throw out the detox medication or bring it back to me. This way there is less chance of a bad outcome.

> ❓ **DID YOU KNOW? Xanax Street Names**
> School buses or gold bars are street names for the long, yellow Xanax 2 mg tablets, which is the highest-strength pill available.

CASE REVISITED: *I see H the next day. He has taken all three doses, and he took an extra dose of 15 mg in the middle of the night. He still has some anxiety, agitation, and cravings, but his tremulousness, sweats, and tachycardia all resolved within 24 hours. At this point I decide to stick with the same dose. I give him a prescription for twenty 30 mg tablets to last him for 3 days, with a plan to reassess at day 1 and day 3.*

Although one might think that I should increase H's dose to cover his remaining psychological symptoms, in fact, given phenobarbital's long half-life of about 100 hours, after only one day his serum levels are still increasing and have not yet reached a steady state.

By day 3, H is doing much better emotionally and physically. He says he is sleeping much better than he had in a long time. We discuss a tapering schedule of decreasing in 15 mg increments every three days. I choose this slower taper because of his moderately severe withdrawal symptoms. He tolerates this well, and eventually he tapers more quickly, dropping a whole tablet at a time. It takes about 3 weeks for him to get completely off. I also start citalopram 10 mg during the second week of treatment for H's anxiety symptoms.

Relapse prevention

One might think that naltrexone or acamprosate would be helpful to prevent sedative relapse, since they are effective for treating addiction to alcohol (aka the liquid sedative). But there is no good evidence—and very little published research—confirming that these meds work for sedative use disorder. While it's possible that future research will support the use of these medications, at this point the best course is to use "supportive" treatments, such as antidepressants and nonaddictive anxiolytics or hypnotics.

Psychosocial treatment involves some combination of 12-step program attendance, psychotherapy, and substance abuse treatment programs,

TABLE 8-1. Characteristics of Commonly Used Sedatives

Generic (Brand)	Tablet or Capsule Strengths*	Average Dosage Range	Equipotent Dose	Onset of Action After Oral Dose	Half-Life (Hours)	Clinical Duration of Action (Hours)	Notes
Alprazolam (Xanax)	0.25 mg, 0.5 mg, 1 mg, 2 mg	1 mg–4 mg/day	0.5 mg	30 minutes	11–16	3–4	Short-acting; high abuse potential
Chlordiazepoxide (Librium)	5 mg, 10 mg, 25 mg	10 mg–200 mg/day	25 mg	1 hour	> 100	4–6	Long-acting; has active metabolites
Clonazepam (Klonopin)	0.5 mg, 1 mg, 2 mg	0.5 mg–2 mg/day	0.5 mg	1 hour	20–80	6–8	Long-acting; has active metabolites
Diazepam (Valium)	2 mg, 5 mg, 10 mg	5 mg–40 mg/day	10 mg	30 minutes	> 100	4–6	Works quickly; long-acting; has active metabolites
Eszopiclone (Lunesta)	1 mg, 2 mg, 3 mg	1 mg–3 mg/day	N/A	30 minutes	6	6–8	Z-drug used as hypnotic; no anxiolytic properties
Lorazepam (Ativan)	0.5 mg, 1 mg, 2 mg	1 mg–4 mg/day	1 mg	30–60 minutes	10–20	4–6	No active metabolites; no P450 metabolism; used in liver disease
Oxazepam (Serax)	10 mg, 15 mg, 30 mg	30 mg–120 mg/day	15 mg	2 hours	8	4–6	No active metabolites; no P450 metabolism; used in liver disease
Phenobarbital	15 mg, 30 mg, 60 mg, 100 mg	60 mg–180 mg/day	N/A	30–60 minutes	79	8+	Long half-life; no active metabolites; not dependent on liver metabolism; used in liver disease
Zaleplon (Sonata)	5 mg, 10 mg	5 mg–20 mg/day	N/A	30 minutes	1	4	Z-drug used as hypnotic; no anxiolytic properties
Zolpidem (Ambien)	5 mg, 10 mg; ER tablet: 6.25 mg, 12.5 mg	5 mg–10 mg/day or 6.25 mg–12.5 mg/day ER	N/A	30 minutes	2.5–3	6–8	Z-drug used as hypnotic; no anxiolytic properties
Zolpidem low dose (Intermezzo)	SL tablet: 1.75 mg, 3.5 mg	1.75 mg–3.5 mg/day	N/A	30 minutes	2.5	4	Z-drug used as hypnotic; no anxiolytic properties

*Only tablet or capsule doses listed, many medications also have orally disintegrating or liquid formulations (For comprehensive information, see Puzantian T and Carlat D. *The Carlat Psychiatry Report Medication Fact Book for Psychiatric Practice*. 3rd ed. Newburyport, MA: Carlat Publishing; 2016) such as intensive outpatient programs. Because there is no specific pharmacotherapy, the focus of behavioral treatment is on developing relapse prevention skills and appropriate coping skills. Anxiety is often a significant component of self-medication with sedatives, so individual and group therapy can be valuable for developing techniques to self-soothe and calm down when dealing with stressful events.

CASE CONCLUSION: *Now that H is not worrying about getting his next Xanax, he is able to think longer-term, and we talk about preventing relapse. I suggest that he see an individual therapist to work on coping skills, since over the years he has relied on Xanax to help him deal with stressful situations. I also recommend a 12-step group, but H isn't interested in that option.*

Self-Test Questions

1. Which of the following receptor systems is activated by lorazepam?
    a. Gamma-aminobutyric acid
    b. Glutamate
    c. N-methyl-d-aspartate
    d. Endocannabinoid

2. A 46-year-old woman has been using a drug several times daily for the past 6 months. She is incarcerated over a weekend for driving with a suspended license. After her second day of incarceration, she develops a tremor in both hands, is diaphoretic and anxious, and keeps talking about hearing mice running around in the walls. Which of the following drugs was this woman most likely taking before her incarceration?
    a. Phencyclidine
    b. Cannabis
    c. Alprazolam
    d. Dimethyltryptamine

3. You are seeing a new patient for generalized anxiety disorder and decide to prescribe an antianxiety antidepressant, citalopram. At the end of the visit, the patient asks if you would prescribe a muscle relaxant for a low-back strain from lifting some boxes the other day, until he can see his

primary care physician. Which of the following medications has a major metabolite that is a sedative?

a. Carisoprodol
b. Lorazepam
c. Methocarbamol
d. Oxazepam

The answer key for these self-test questions is on page 233.

Note: If you purchased CME credit with this book, your CME post-test can be accessed when you are logged in at www.thecarlatreport.com/AddictionGuide. Please keep in mind that the question and answer order for that CME post-test are different than what you see in these self-test study questions.

CHAPTER 9

Nicotine

**"Giving up smoking is the easiest thing in the world.
I know because I've done it thousands of times."**
Mark Twain

TAKE HOME POINTS

- Nicotine is similar to stimulants because it enhances alertness, and it also causes feelings of relaxation.
- Smoking becomes associated with many activities throughout the day, which can trigger cravings that lead to relapse.
- Electronic cigarettes are less harmful than tobacco cigarettes, but they are not completely safe and can also cause nicotine addiction.
- Behavioral techniques are the mainstay of smoking cessation treatment.
- Pharmacotherapy for nicotine use disorder includes nicotine replacement therapy, Chantix, and Zyban.
- Most smokers require multiple quit attempts before they are successful, so continue to encourage patients to try again.

CASE VIGNETTE: *I first met Y when she was being treated for depression, but she was not interested in quitting smoking then. She was a 42-year-old female who was smoking 1 pack per day and had previously smoked up to 1.5 packs per day. She had tried to quit smoking multiple times on her own, and had also tried the nicotine patch. However, she would resume smoking due to anxiety and irritability, either without using the patch or several weeks after stopping it.*

ESSENTIALS OF NICOTINE

The gateway theory of addiction describes a sequence and progression of addictive substance use, from tobacco and alcohol to cannabis, then to other illicit drugs like heroin and cocaine. Cigarettes are a powerful gateway drug to diverse illegal drugs, especially among adolescents.

Most U.S. adolescents will experiment with tobacco before age 18, and many will develop a tobacco use disorder by late adolescence. Adolescents tend to overestimate their peers' use of tobacco products, and peer group imitation is a significant driver of early tobacco use. Each year, around 70% of tobacco cigarette smokers say they want to quit, and over half of them make a quit attempt. Unfortunately, relapse rates are very high, from 60% to 90% within the first year.

Immediate effects

Nicotine is one of about 4,000 chemicals present in cigarette smoke, but it is the most active psychologically and is responsible for the addictive properties of smoking. When smoked, the nicotine is quickly absorbed by the lung's alveoli, reaching the brain within seconds of the first puff. The chemical appears to work by stimulating acetylcholine receptors that are attached to dopamine neurons, which rapidly release dopamine to produce the nicotine buzz. (These receptors are sometimes confusingly called "nicotinic receptors," because they are a subclass of acetylcholine receptors that are stimulated by nicotine.) The effects diminish quickly, leading users to want another hit to replicate the feeling. With regular use, receptor sites are down-regulated, resulting in the smoker needing more nicotine to produce the same effects.

The effects of nicotine are similar to the effects of stronger stimulants such as cocaine and amphetamines. Nicotine enhances alertness and focus, but also causes muscle relaxation. As with stimulants, memories of the pleasurable effects are associated with whatever is going on at the time of tobacco use. Typical times for smoking—such as in the car, while talking on the telephone, with a cup of coffee, after a good meal, or after sex—become strongly associated with the use of nicotine and its pleasurable effects. These then become triggers to smoke again. These are called *cue cravings* or *trigger cravings*, and are a large part of the day-to-day habit of smoking.

Another effect of nicotine is appetite suppression, also similar to more potent stimulants. This is one reason cigarettes are popular for weight control among teenage girls.

Nicotine's immediate physiologic effects include mild tachycardia.

Long-term effects

Nicotine's dangers in terms of cancer and heart disease risk are well known. Additionally, from a psychiatric perspective, nicotine is a stimulant and can worsen anxiety and mood disorders. Since it is an inducer of the 1A2 P450 metabolic enzyme, it can complicate dosing of medications, most notably olanzapine and clozapine.

Withdrawal syndrome

Nicotine withdrawal does not have obvious physical symptoms, but rather subjective effects such as reduced alertness, irritability, and headache. This is not as pronounced as the crash from stimulants such as cocaine or methamphetamine, but it is uncomfortable and reduces productivity. The withdrawal syndrome lasts for 7–10 days, then the symptoms drop off sharply and gradually improve from that point. In addition to the withdrawal symptoms, cravings are prominent and can be intense. Fortunately, an episode of acute craving is fairly short, usually only about 20 minutes. If a patient can hold out that long, the craving will subside. Most smokers who are trying to quit will relapse within a few days due to withdrawal symptoms and cravings.

Electronic cigarettes

Electronic nicotine delivery systems, or "e-cigarettes," generally consist of a power source (usually a battery, but adapters can draw power from an electrical outlet, a car's electrical outlet, or a computer USB port) and heating element (commonly referred to as an atomizer) that vaporizes a solution (known as "e-liquid" or "e-juice"). The user inhales the vapor, which is called "vaping" instead of smoking. E-liquids contain propylene glycol and/or vegetable glycerin, flavorings, and nicotine. Ask patients specifically about their use of electronic cigarettes in addition to tobacco cigarettes, since patients may not consider them to be a "tobacco product."

E-cigarettes may have the potential for less physical harm compared to tobacco, since they do not deliver carbon monoxide and they expose the user to fewer carcinogens. However, they do deliver nicotine, which is addictive. They also expose the user to other chemicals, pollens, and impurities. When asked whether e-cigarettes are safer than tobacco cigarettes, my response is that e-cigarettes are generally safer than tobacco, but not as safe as air.

E-cigarettes are neither designed nor marketed as smoking cessation devices. Their original purpose was to provide a way for users to get around smoking bans in public places (buildings, restaurants, airplanes) by allowing them to vape nicotine instead of exposing others to secondhand tobacco smoke. Some people have tried to quit smoking by using e-cigarettes, and clinical trials have shown that e-cigarettes can be fairly effective in helping smokers cut down or cease tobacco use. Personally, I do not recommend e-cigarettes to my patients for smoking cessation, since there are several other more successful options available.

Even if people use e-cigarettes to quit smoking tobacco, there are risks associated with these devices. As with other drugs of abuse, e-cigarette users may escalate their dose of nicotine due to physical tolerance. The voltage of newer types of e-cigarettes can be adjusted by the user, and higher voltage increases the nicotine yield of the vapor. Users may also tamper with the e-cigarette delivery system to provide larger doses of nicotine, or change to a higher nicotine concentration in the e-liquid. Bottles containing e-liquid to refill e-cigarette cartridges may contain up to 720 mg of nicotine—if ingested, this is not only toxic, but potentially fatal.

ASSESSMENT

To officially diagnose tobacco use disorder, a "problematic pattern" of tobacco use must be established, leading to "significant distress" which lasts at least 12 months. DSM-5 lists 11 criteria, which are the same for other substances; the severity guidelines are the same as well (meeting at least 2 criteria is mild, 4 is moderate, and 6 is severe). First, assess what your patients are ingesting, how much they're ingesting, and how addicted they are. Answering these questions will help you come up with the best method of attacking the problem.

1. Determine the daily nicotine load. Ask about packs per day of cigarettes, but make sure to ask about e-cigarettes, chewing tobacco, and hookah pipes, all of which are increasingly popular. While the nicotine content

of the average cigarette is pretty standard (1 mg), it's harder to figure out how much your patients are getting through other options. E-cigarettes used to deliver less nicotine than tobacco cigarettes, but that's no longer always true. For chewing tobacco, one pouch is generally the equivalent of about a quarter of a pack of cigarettes. Ask, "How many times do you refill your e-cigarette cartridge?" "How many packets of chewing tobacco do you go through per day?"

2. Determine the usage pattern. Get a feel for the patient's degree of tolerance and addiction. Ask, "When do you have your first cigarette of the day?" If the patient wakes up, takes a shower, has breakfast, and then lights up, that's less concerning than a patient who shuts off the alarm with one hand and lights a cigarette with the other. Ask, "Do you smoke when you're sick?" Those who do are more physically dependent. A good resource is the Fagerström test (see Appendix), which has a list of questions you can ask to assess your patient's degree of tolerance.

3. Has a quit method worked for the patient in the past—or *not* worked? You might hear things like, "I tried the patch but it gave me nightmares," or "I did the best when I quit cold turkey." The responses you receive will help guide your patient's treatment.

Key questions to ask:

- What activities have you given up to smoke? These can be school, work, social, or other fun activities.
- Do you have cravings to smoke? How often? What sets off your cravings?
- Have there been times when you smoked more than you intended?
- When do you smoke the most? This can be a time, place, or activity.
- Tell me about times when you have tried to cut down or quit smoking.

CASE REVISITED: *Y had her first cigarette of the day with her morning coffee, after brushing her teeth but before breakfast and a shower. She smoked 20 cigarettes (1 pack) throughout the day. She smoked several in the morning in the house and in her car on the way to work, then took several smoke breaks while at work, including on her lunch break; this also helped her not eat so much at lunch. When her workplace first banned smoking several years ago, she made her first serious quit attempt with the nicotine patch, but was unsuccessful. Later quit attempts were often thwarted by stress at work because she liked the relaxing feeling a cigarette* *gave her during the day. Y bought some disposable electronic cigarettes last year, but when she tried vaping these at work, she didn't get the immediate feeling of relaxation that she was used to, and the flavor was different from her usual brand of tobacco cigarettes.*

TREATMENT

Non-pharmacologic treatment

Studies have shown that simply advising your patients to quit along with agreeing on a quit date can be helpful. Even more effective are behavioral therapy and motivational interviewing—but that may not be available to certain patients, depending on where they live and what kind of insurance they have (see Chapter 4 for information on motivational interviewing). Fortunately, there are several free resources, some of which are paid for by manufacturers of smoking cessation treatments. The best portal is the phone number 1-800-QUIT-NOW, and there are various affiliated websites. One is www.smokefree.gov, maintained by the U.S. Department of Health and Human Services. Patients can get diaries and calendars to support their efforts, and they can sign up for a phone call or text message on their quit date, as well as follow-up calls or texts. The site also has information on using diaries and calendars to support quitting efforts. While these programs are designed to be used in conjunction with nicotine replacement therapy or other pharmacologic treatment, they are helpful for anyone.

DOCTOR/PATIENT DIALOGUE: Motivational Interviewing to Persuade a Patient to Quit

Doctor: Have you thought about quitting smoking?

Patient: Smoking relaxes me.

Doctor: Yes, it can help people relax. What else do you like about smoking?

Patient: Like? No doc has asked me that before. Let's see . . . I like taking a break during the day. I like talking with people who are also outside smoking. That first cigarette of the day is the best. I used to look pretty cool lighting up and puffing away in front of my friends, but that got kind of old after a while.

Doctor: So the excuse to take a break during the workday is good, and the first cigarette of the day is the best one, but lighting up isn't as cool now as it used to be. Is anything else not as much fun as it used to be?

Patient: Well, it costs real money, that's for sure. And going outside all the time gets old, too. If I knock over an ashtray in the house, cleaning it up is a pain. I also don't like that I can't give it up, even for a while. But if I didn't have my cigarettes, I couldn't make it through my day.

Doctor: So it's expensive, it takes some time in your day away from other things, and cleaning up is a hassle. Anything else?

Patient: My mother quit when she was younger, so she's on my case about me smoking. I swear, she brings it up all the time. I've taken to hiding the ashtrays when she comes to visit, and I sneak out of my own house to take a drag, just to avoid the hassle.

Doctor: So your mother would support you if you would try to quit, and she would be proud of you if you did?

Patient: I guess so.

Doctor: That sounds like something to think about.

Patient: Yeah, I'm sure I'll try to quit again someday. I'm not ready now.

Doctor: You're right; it's worth thinking about quitting again. You might find you can relax without a cigarette. It might even help your depression.

Patient: I suppose so. I'll think about it—especially if it could help my depression.

Doctor: Is it all right if I ask about that at our next visit?

Patient: Okay. I'll let you know.

Pharmacologic treatment

Nicotine replacement therapy (NRT)

NRT supplies an alternative source of nicotine to help your patients decrease and ultimately quit smoking. I recommend starting with NRT before moving to bupropion or varenicline, because it's widely available and readily acceptable to most smokers.

Which NRT to choose? There are lots of options, but generally you should start with the patch, because it delivers a constant nicotine level throughout the day, hopefully preventing episodes of craving. (For really light smokers, you can start with nicotine gum—see below.) Patches used to be expensive, but prices have come down as more chain pharmacies have created their own products. At this point, a month's supply will generally cost about $1 per day.

Which dose of the patch should you prescribe? It depends on your patient's current nicotine consumption. A typical pack-per-day smoker is consuming about 20 mg of nicotine per day, so in this case you would prescribe the 21 mg patch. If the patient smokes 2 packs per day, 2 patches may be needed, but this (and even lesser doses) may be too much, and some patients will simply discontinue the patch if they have adverse effects. It's recommended to counsel patients that they can reduce the dose if needed.

I tell patients to apply the patch at the same time each day, usually in the morning. One potential exception is the smoker who wakes up with a strong craving to smoke. Such patients can try applying the patch close to bedtime, following the theory that the residual morning nicotine will prevent their initial craving. A common problem with nighttime administration is vivid dreams or nightmares, so warn your patient: "You might notice some funky dreams."

In terms of where to place the patch, tell your patient to start by placing it just above the heart (the upper anterior chest), then the next day move it left to the upper arm, then the left upper back, right upper back, right shoulder, right chest, and finally back above the heart. This rotation helps prevent skin irritation due to the adhesive. If there is any irritation, 0.5% cortisone cream helps. Usually no shaving is required. Swimming with the patch is fine, and patients who think they'll be embarrassed by wearing a patch on the beach can be reassured that patches are clear now and pretty hard to spot.

Have your patients stay on the initial dose for 4–6 weeks, then use the next-lower strength for 4 weeks, and so on. Some patients need a longer taper—for example, they may need 3 months on the initial dose, and then a very slow taper thereafter. Advise patients not to smoke while taking the patch, but let's face it—some will. With this in mind, be realistic and tell them that if they do smoke, they may develop nausea, which is the first symptom of nicotine toxicity.

🔍 NICOTINE PATCH—AT A GLANCE	
Indication	Tobacco cessation
Dosages available	7 mg, 14 mg, 21 mg
Target dose	Start 14 mg–21 mg daily, then gradually taper over several weeks
Comments	Several other forms of NRT are available, including gum, lozenge, and spray

Combination NRT

Some patients find that they have cravings throughout the day even while using the patch—if so, recommend one of the short-acting NRT agents, such as the gum, lozenge, or spray, in combination with the patch. In fact, light smokers may do well starting with one of these agents and skipping the patch entirely.

A word on nicotine gum: Its chewing technique is different from regular gum. Patients should start by chewing a few times to activate the release of the nicotine; they'll know it's releasing because the gum will start tasting bad and peppery. At that point, they should park it between the cheek and the gums, and switch sides every several minutes or so. One piece of gum releases a total of either 2 mg or 4 mg of nicotine, and it lasts about 30 minutes.

While the gum is the most popular short-acting treatment, some patients will prefer other options, such as the lozenge or the spray. The lozenge is easy to use—patients just pop one in like a piece of hard candy when they have the urge to smoke. Nicotine nasal spray is available by prescription and involves frequent dosing of small amounts of nicotine. Its use is limited to six months to prevent development of physical dependence on nicotine (obviously counterproductive given the goal of tobacco cessation).

Varenicline (Chantix)

Chantix acts as a partial agonist at nicotinic receptors, so its mechanism is physiologically closer to nicotine—which is our rationale for choosing it over other medications, such as bupropion. Some patients will move on to Chantix after an unsuccessful trial of NRT, but others want to start with the pill right away, which is reasonable.

While Chantix's manufacturer has a dosing recommendation, different clinicians have their own preferences based on experience. I start patients with 0.5 mg per day for 7–10 days, at which point they should stop smoking and increase to 1 mg BID, then continue at that dose for 3 months. However, a recent study found that patients don't have to quit that soon after starting Chantix to respond to the drug. In the study, smokers were asked to reduce their smoking gradually over 3 months while taking Chantix, and their long-term abstinence rates were robust—27% at one year vs. 9.9% on placebo (Ebbert et al, 2015). This is good news because some patients panic when told they have to try quitting in a week.

Chantix's potential psychiatric side effects have been widely covered, but in my opinion, they're overblown. A recent meta-analysis of 39 randomized controlled trials covering 10,761 patients found that there was no difference between Chantix and placebo in rates of depression, suicidal ideation, or aggression (Thomas et al, 2015). However, Chantix did cause more insomnia and abnormal dreams in these studies, which jibes with my experience. Tell patients about the possibility of vivid dreams and nightmares (though nightmares aren't very common). If this is a problem, have them take the pills in the morning.

🔍 VARENICLINE (CHANTIX)—AT A GLANCE	
Indication	Tobacco cessation
Dosages available	0.5 mg, 1 mg
Target dose	1 mg twice daily

Bupropion (Wellbutrin, Zyban)

One large study reported that bupropion SR led to a 23% one-year quit rate vs. 12% for placebo (Hurt, 1997). While the manufacturer recommends starting at 150 mg per day for 3 days then increasing to 150 mg BID, studies have shown that continuing with 150 mg/day is just as effective as the higher dose—and has fewer side effects.

Most psychiatric prescribers are quite familiar with bupropion's common side effects of insomnia and anxiety. A potentially good side effect is weight

🔍 BUPROPION (WELLBUTRIN, ZYBAN)—AT A GLANCE	
Indications	Major depression, SAD, tobacco cessation
Dosages available	75 mg, 100 mg, 150 mg, 200 mg
Target dose	300 mg for smoking cessation

TABLE 9-1. Tobacco Cessation Drugs

Product	Dose	Side Effects
Nicotine patch	7 mg, 14 mg, 21 mg/day, depending on nicotine use	Application site reactions
Nicotine gum	2 mg–4 mg every 1–2 hours as needed	Headache, indigestion, nausea
Nicotine lozenge	2 mg–4 mg every 1–2 hours as needed	Headache, indigestion, nausea
Varenicline (Chantix)	Start 0.5 mg/day, increase to 1 mg twice daily	Insomnia, vivid dreams
Bupropion (Wellbutrin, Zyban)	150 mg, either once or twice daily	Tremor, insomnia, weight loss
Nortriptyline (off-label)	Start 25 mg daily, increase to 75 mg–100 mg daily	Sedation, dry mouth, constipation
Clonidine (off-label)	Start 0.1 mg daily, increase to maximum of 0.75 mg total daily	Hypotension, sedation, dry mouth

loss, since people trying to quit smoking often substitute food for cigarettes. Note that bupropion is contraindicated in patients with a seizure disorder or with a history of bulimia or anorexia nervosa.

Off-label meds

Two medications, nortriptyline and clonidine, are effective second-line agents for smoking cessation, though this is an off-label use for both. Nortriptyline is usually started at 25 mg daily 10–28 days before the quit date, then gradually increased to 75 mg–100 mg daily. Treat for 3 months at this dose; the treatment can be extended to a total of 6 months depending on response. Nortriptyline should be tapered off instead of stopped abruptly due to possibility of withdrawal effects. Clonidine is dosed starting with 0.1 mg daily, then increased gradually as tolerated by 0.1 mg/day to a 0.15 mg–0.75 mg total daily dose. Clonidine should also be tapered off to avoid rebound effects.

CASE REVISITED: *Since Y had tried nicotine replacement therapy without much success, I recommended varenicline. I also recommended nicotine lozenges to use if she had cravings that she could not overcome with distraction techniques. I gave her information on 1-800-QUIT-NOW and smokefree.gov, and I encouraged her to access the online behavioral program that came with her varenicline prescription. Finally, I encouraged*

Y to let her coworkers and friends know about her quit attempt, so that nonsmokers could offer her support and her coworkers would not try to tempt her back into smoking.

QUITTING AND PREVENTING RELAPSE

Unfortunately, most patients relapse, even with the fanciest of meds and behavioral therapy; let them know that there's no shame in failing to quit. I say things like, "You may have to try this several times—and that's okay." Often I'll invoke the Mark Twain quote that leads off this chapter.

The first week after quitting is the hardest in terms of craving. A typical smoker gets about 10 puffs out of a cigarette, meaning that a pack-per-day smoker gets 200 doses of nicotine over the course of a day. That's a lot of habituation and reinforcement the patient must overcome. Triggers for craving are everywhere—seeing the ashtray, having coffee, having a drink, going to the corner store, etc. Distraction techniques can work well, because nicotine cravings generally only last 10–20 minutes. Patients can do things like drink a large glass of cold water or play a video game to get their minds off the urge.

I recommend warning patients that they are likely to cough temporarily after they quit—this is a normal response as the cilia of the lungs "wake up" and get rid of mucus. If not alerted to this, some patients will worry unnecessarily.

In my experience, even with the high rate of relapse, patients who are willing to stick it out with you over time will have at least a 50% chance of prolonged abstinence.

Here are some practical tips for successful quitting and relapse prevention.

- **Set a quit date.** Have the patient set a significant quit date, such as a birthday or anniversary, to enhance motivation. Conversely, a quit date can be set during a time when the patient has less stress and can deal with the difficulties of a quit attempt. Before setting a quit date, I recommend patients immediately start gradually reducing their daily number of cigarettes. This way, they will be smoking less before they stop completely, which can help with the severity of early nicotine withdrawal symptoms. They will also start to get used to those symptoms, at least to a degree.

- **Tell friends and family.** If other people know the patient is quitting, they can provide support. Family, friends, or coworkers can also help keep the patient accountable—if the patient lights up a cigarette around them, they can say, "I thought you were quitting!"
- **Have everyone try to quit together.** If the patient has a partner or roommate who is a smoker, the patient is much more likely to relapse. If both try to quit, they can support one another and are much more likely to be successful.
- **Reduce the prevalence of cigarettes.** Here are a few ways:
  - *Limit smoking to outside the home.* This helps the patient to think twice about automatically lighting up. It makes smoking intentionally less convenient. If smoking an individual cigarette becomes more of a hassle, the patient is more likely to say, "Forget it; I'll just smoke later."
  - *Get rid of all but one ashtray in the home.* Then get rid of the last ashtray on the quit date.
  - *Switch to a different brand of cigarettes.* The difference in taste from a new brand can help reduce the number of cigarettes smoked per day and remind patients that they are not supposed to be smoking as much. However, switching to "light" (lower-nicotine) cigarettes doesn't work—patients just smoke more cigarettes to make up the difference.

CASE CONCLUSION: *Y set her quit date for her nephew's high school graduation. She took up most of the behavioral strategies I suggested, including getting rid of ashtrays and smoking only on her back patio. She started varenicline 10 days before her quit date and signed up for the manufacturer's behavioral program, which included an app for her smartphone.*

Y was on varenicline for 3 months and only smoked a few cigarettes during that time, primarily due to stress from deadlines at work. She did not have any worsening of depression, nor any suicidal ideation while taking varenicline. She found the lozenges were helpful for cravings at first, but didn't use them for long because she didn't want to spend the money for them. Due to ongoing cravings, she chose to continue varenicline for another 3 months. By the end of that time, Y was no longer smoking and felt confident in her ability to remain abstinent. She appreciated the extra money she had available and found that she was more productive at work, which was a pleasant surprise.

Self-Test Questions

1. A 55-year-old woman who is attempting to quit smoking presents with a rash on her arm where she places her nicotine patches. She has had the rash for 3 days and reports that it is red and itchy. She started using a nicotine 21 mg daily patch 3 weeks ago and has not smoked since then. The patient feels well otherwise and has no cravings for tobacco. Physical examination shows an area of erythema underneath her patch with no swelling or skin breakdown. Which of the following is the most appropriate next step in management?
    a. Discontinue the nicotine patch and encourage her to continue to abstain from tobacco
    b. Discontinue the nicotine patch and start varenicline
    c. Rotate the patch to a different site when changing patches, and monitor the rash
    d. Switch to a nicotine patch with a lower dosage

2. A 45-year-old woman with bipolar disorder is admitted to an inpatient treatment program because of a 2-week history of an acute exacerbation of mania. The patient has smoked 1.5 packs of cigarettes daily for the past 25 years. The hospital prohibits cigarette smoking on its grounds. Which of the following is the most appropriate pharmacotherapy to manage tobacco use disorder in this patient?
    a. Nicotine transdermal patch 14 mg daily
    b. Nicotine transdermal patch 21 mg daily
    c. Oral bupropion SR 150 mg twice daily
    d. Oral varenicline 1 mg twice daily

3. A 58-year-old man has tried multiple times to quit smoking—changing cigarette brands, using nicotine patches, and even undergoing hypnosis—with no success. You suggest that a combination treatment approach has been shown to improve smoking cessation outcomes. Which of the following has been shown to improve rates of smoking cessation when combined with nicotine replacement therapy?
    a. Biofeedback
    b. Clonidine
    c. Behavioral program
    d. Acupuncture

The answer key for these self-test questions is on page 233.

Note: If you purchased CME credit with this book, your CME post-test can be accessed when you are logged in at www.thecarlatreport.com/AddictionGuide. Please keep in mind that the question and answer order for that CME post-test are different than what you see in these self-test study questions.

CHAPTER 10

Cannabis

"So many writers make dope glamorous; a form of romantic transgression, or world-weariness, or poetic sensitivity, or hipness. Mainly it's the stuff of ritualistic communion among inarticulate bores."
Leonard Michaels

TAKE HOME POINTS

- The psychoactive component of cannabis is THC, and THC content varies widely.
- Long-term use can cause chronic cannabis syndrome, impacting school and career performance and potentially aggravating anxiety, depression, and psychosis.
- Evidence-based medical uses for cannabis are few: intractable nausea, AIDS wasting syndrome, and pain due to neurological spasticity.
- Withdrawal from heavy use can cause nausea, irritability, and insomnia.
- There is no effective medication to treat marijuana use disorder.

CASE VIGNETTE: *J, a 23-year-old male, is referred to me by another psychiatrist. He had started using marijuana at age 13, and began using regularly (several times a week) when he was 18. He had enrolled at a state university, but dropped out after two years. He had suffered anxiety problems, including panic attacks, since high school, and the anxiety had worsened over the past year. J sought treatment for the anxiety through a local mental health clinic, and once his long history of cannabis use was disclosed, the treating psychiatrist referred J to me to help with reducing his use and to evaluate whether it was causing the anxiety.*

ESSENTIALS OF CANNABIS

Cannabis derives from the cannabis sativa plant, a variety of hemp that has been cultivated for much of human history. The leaves can be smoked, though the flowering tops and buds are more potent; a resin from the plant can also be concentrated into hash or hash oil. The main psychoactive component is delta-9-tetrahydrocannabinol (THC), which is one of many cannabinoids in the plant.

THC activates cannabinoid receptors in the brain. Two subtypes have been identified: Type 1 is predominant in the brain and is responsible for most of cannabis' psychoactive properties; type 2 is in the periphery, especially in white blood cells, and has effects on the immune system. There are also some endogenous cannabinoids (called endocannabinoids), such as anandamide, which is named after the Sanskrit word "ananda," meaning bliss. It's not clear why we have this endocannabinoid system, but it is ubiquitous throughout the central nervous system and appears to be part of the normal regulation of various functions, including memory, pain sensation, mood, and appetite (Ligresti et al, 2016).

Immediate effects

Cannabis' immediate effects are euphoria, distortion of one's sense of time, and a feeling of enhanced perception of things like colors and music. Some people experience hallucinations and anxiety, and drowsiness is common. The ability to form new memories is impaired during intoxication, though the ability to recall old memories is not affected. Immediate physiological effects include peripheral vasodilation (responsible for users' bloodshot eyes, which is caused by swelling of blood vessels in the sclera, or conjunctival injection) and elevated heart rate (to some degree, this is also caused by peripheral vasodilation).

Overdoses lead to panic attacks, psychotic symptoms, palpitations and tachycardia, and occasionally shortness of breath and chest pain.

Long-term effects

Chronic cannabis syndrome, formerly known as amotivational syndrome, results from long-term regular use of cannabis—especially use during adolescence, which is a vulnerable time for the developing brain. When the immature endocannabinoid system is repeatedly exposed to THC, there

> **FUN FACT: An Anti-Munchies Drug**
>
> It's well known that cannabis causes increased appe-
> tite, otherwise known as the munchies. Pharmaceuti-
> cal companies have taken advantage of this property. For example,
> the synthetic THC agent dronabinol (Marinol) is FDA-approved for
> appetite restoration in AIDS wasting syndrome. Scientists have also
> developed cannabinoid receptor antagonists as potential weight
> loss agents, and in 2006, Sanofi Aventis launched a specific CB-1
> antagonist called rimonabant (brand name Acomplia) (Pi-Sunyer
> et al, 2006). Acomplia was first sold in Great Britain, with plans for
> eventual FDA approval, but reports of depression and suicide as
> apparent side effects caused it to be withdrawn from all markets.

can be long-term subtle effects on learning and adaptation. This may be caused by interference with the normal process of neural pruning during adolescence (Lubman et al, 2015).

Chronic cannabis syndrome has two components: reduction in the ability to process and remember new information and skills, and lessened motivation for achievement in general. This can hinder educational and career trajectories, causing a user's IQ to not meet that of age-matched peers.

In addition to these long-term cognitive effects, cannabis can worsen a range of mental psychiatric symptoms. These include anxiety, with an increased frequency and intensity of panic attacks, as well as depression. Most alarmingly, there is an association between early cannabis use and development of schizophrenia and other psychotic disorders. The risk for psychosis increases with younger age of initiation and a family history of any psychotic disorder or major mental health disorder. A recent review estimated that chronic cannabis use is associated with a twofold increase in risk of developing schizophrenia; however, the causal link is not established (Gage et al, 2016).

Physical effects

Lungs. Inhaling smoke from any source exposes the lungs to potentially toxic material, such as particulate matter or carcinogens. It can worsen asthma and potentially cause chronic obstructive pulmonary disease. Unlike tobacco cigarettes, cannabis joints do not have filters, allowing more contaminants to enter the lungs. On the other hand, people generally smoke fewer joints than tobacco cigarettes, somewhat mitigating this problem.

Heart. Regardless of how it is ingested, cannabis can raise the risk of heart attacks in people with preexisting ischemic heart disease. The mechanism for this risk is cannabis-induced tachycardia, which raises myocardial oxygen demand. This risk is greatest within the first 20 minutes of starting use.

Immune system. Regular cannabis use can reduce immune function, which is most problematic in those who are immunosuppressed, such as people with HIV. Patients who use cannabis during or immediately after receiving chemotherapy for cancer are at risk. Not only can cannabis further reduce immune function, but processing of cannabis is not regulated by the FDA—unlike dronabinol, which is FDA-approved for nausea due to chemotherapy—so cannabis products may contain fungi (especially Aspergillis) and other microorganisms that can lead to opportunistic infections during periods of immunosuppression.

Fertility. Cannabis can reduce fertility in both men and women. It lowers sperm counts in men, and long-term or heavy use can lead to irregular menstrual cycles in women.

Withdrawal

Cannabis withdrawal syndrome is well established and is more psychological than physiological. Symptoms include depression, irritability, appetite suppression, and headaches. In heavy users, there may be diarrhea and other intestinal discomfort, including nausea and vomiting. Cannabis withdrawal symptoms may last 3–7 days, depending on the amount of prior use.

A GUIDE TO CANNABIS PRODUCTS

As cannabis has become legal in many parts of the country, the cannabis industry has grown and the products available have multiplied. As a practitioner, you should be familiar with the major types of products, because they vary significantly in potency, duration of action, and safety. Here is a quick primer of the current state of cannabis products (see Table 10-1 for a quick reference).

Smoked products. The most common and familiar form of cannabis products are smokable joints or blunts, although water pipes and vaporizers are

TABLE 10-1. Available Cannabis Products

Product	Description	Notes
Smoked products (aka joint)	Cannabis flowers, leaves, and/or buds rolled in thin paper and smoked like a tobacco cigarette	Simplest and most common way to use cannabis
Blunt	Cannabis rolled with tobacco in a cigar	
Skunk	Cannabis plant bred with higher THC concentration	British slang term
Water pipe (aka bong or hookah)	Device to filter smoke through water during the smoking process	Paraphernalia for smoking; illegal in some states
Vaporizer	Type of device that uses a battery to heat and vaporize cannabis for inhalation	Paraphernalia for smoking; illegal in some states (an e-cigarette is a small, portable vaporizer)
Hash oil	Cannabis plant matter soaked in a chemical solvent to extract concentrated THC resin	Can be smoked, vaped, or ingested orally
Edibles	Wide variety of food products infused with hash oil and consumed orally	Baked goods and candies; may have 5 mg–100 mg of THC per product
Shatter (aka butane honey oil, dab, or wax)	THC resin extracted from cannabis plant with butane as the solvent	Flammable; may explode during manufacturing or storage

also used. In the 1960s and 1970s, the THC content in cultivated cannabis plants was in the low single digits. However, newer strains have THC levels in the 10%–20% range. There are also other varieties called "skunk," which are much more potent.

Hash oils. These are typically ingested using electronic vapor delivery devices, essentially identical to e-cigarettes (see Chapter 9 for details). The devices and hash oil e-liquids are sold legally in certain states. Many e-cigarettes with refillable e-liquid tanks can also be used to vape hash oil, making it potentially difficult to determine whether someone is vaping nicotine or cannabis.

Edibles. In addition to the familiar pot brownies, now there are cannabis-containing cookies and cupcakes, as well as hash oil–infused chocolate candy

> ### ODD FACT: Cannabis Hyperemesis Syndrome
>
> Few people have heard of an unusual syndrome that sometimes occurs with heavy cannabis use: Patients will experience severe nausea and vomiting. This is particularly strange because one of THC's therapeutic effects is *reducing* nausea, rather than triggering it. Cessation of cannabis use will stop the nausea, and long hot baths and showers provide significant relief, which is a clinical clue to diagnosis of this rare syndrome. With more widespread use of cannabis products as more U.S. states legalize their possession, cannabis hyperemesis may become more common.

bars, gummy bears, and lollipops. Users can even add raw cannabis plant material to butter at home and simmer it to make cannabis-infused butter, also known as "cannabutter." In states where they are legal, cannabis-infused products must carry a label disclosing the amount of cannabis they contain.

Compared to smoked cannabis, edibles have slower onset of action and longer duration. Whereas smoked cannabis takes effect immediately and lasts about 3 hours, edibles have a delayed onset of an hour or so, and can last 8 hours or more. Portion control is difficult, and in some cases dangerous, particularly when there are children around. A cannabis chocolate bar, for example, may be one dose per square, but someone who mistakenly eats the entire bar would experience paranoia, hallucinations, and problems with coordination.

Synthetic cannabinoids. These versions of cannabis were originally developed at university and drug company labs, initially for research into developing medications. Eventually, these compounds were coopted by clandestine chemists to create designer drugs such as spice, K2, and kush, all of which are much more powerful than natural cannabis. There is more information on these substances in Chapter 13.

ASSESSMENT

Cannabis users often do not have insight about how the drug has affected their lives. A common issue in young users is poor performance at school or jobs. I'll ask something like, "Two years ago, where did you see yourself in terms of what you would achieve?" They might say, "I would have had a job or gone to college." Then we discuss how things got delayed, and I'll ask, "Why did your life go off track? What were you doing instead?" Cannabis is often the explanation, and we engage in that discussion.

In terms of school, cannabis can impair progress in two interconnected ways: It decreases the motivation to study, but it also decreases users' comprehension and memory of what they are studying. Some will attribute their lack of attention in class to not liking the course, or they might say they were spending time doing other things besides studying. I point out one of the things they were doing was using marijuana.

It can be difficult to know how much THC patients are consuming because there are so many strains. One way to get a rough idea is to ask how much they are spending on their habit per day or per week. For example, a "dime bag" refers to a $10 bag, and a "quarter" is a $25 bag. The amount of cannabis in these bags varies, but commonly a dime bag will contain about 1 gram, which might be enough for a couple of joints.

Ask about psychiatric symptoms, especially anxiety and hallucinations. Hallucinatory experiences are more common among older users and with large amounts of cannabis. If a patient has an established anxiety disorder, look for the relationship between cannabis use and those symptoms.

CASE REVISITED: *J smokes 6 to 10 joints most days. His use has escalated, and he has been through several cycles of withdrawal, with symptoms of nausea, anxiety, and irritability. He craves cannabis, restricts his relationships to regular cannabis users, has driven under the influence, and was once arrested for possession. I diagnose him with severe cannabis use disorder, as well as substance-induced anxiety disorder.*

TREATMENT

Since there is no pharmacotherapy helpful in reducing cannabis use, treatment involves a combination of motivational interviewing, help with detox, and behavioral strategies.

Motivational interviewing: Discussing pros and cons of cannabis with your patients

Cannabis is unique among substances of abuse in that its legal status is in flux, and the legalization movement has provided users with various rationales to defend their use. Regardless of whether you believe cannabis has benefits, you should be ready to have informed discussions with your patients about the issue. Here are some typical statements regarding cannabis use that you may hear from your patients, followed by my take on these issues and how I usually discuss them with patients.

"I use marijuana as medical treatment." As of this writing, medical marijuana is legal in 28 states. How is medical marijuana different from dronabinol, which has long been legal to prescribe throughout the U.S.? Dronabinol is a highly regulated compound that is purified THC. Medical marijuana, by contrast, refers to a wide range of products, most of which have little regulation or quality control, although this situation may improve as states implement medical marijuana legislation.

There is evidence for cannabis' effectiveness in a small number of conditions, including intractable nausea from cancer chemotherapy and appetite enhancement for AIDS wasting syndrome, the two indications for which dronabinol has FDA approval. It is also used off-label for pain management, muscle spasms, glaucoma, and multiple sclerosis. However, even for these conditions, cannabis is considered at best second-line treatment.

Scientific evidence does not support efficacy of cannabis for psychiatric illnesses. In practice, when patients are using cannabis, it is more difficult to gauge whether the medication you are prescribing (such as an antidepressant or benzodiazepine) is having a therapeutic effect.

"Many successful people get high." Presidents, CEOs, journalists, movie stars—it's not hard to identify prominent and successful people who have used cannabis. Some patients believe this means there is no harm in using it. But for all the success stories, there are many famous people (Lindsay Lohan, Willie Nelson, Macaulay Culkin) who have ongoing and public problems caused by their addiction. Many celebrities have a good deal of money and a team of high-powered lawyers to help them avoid jail or large fines. Your patients probably don't.

"I'm not addicted; I'm using it recreationally." Some patients describe their cannabis use as casual and recreational, which may be true, but if they are seeking psychiatric treatment, you should be skeptical of how benign that use really is. In these cases, I'll use my standard motivational interviewing techniques to explore whether patients are, in fact, ambivalent about their use. I'll ask, "What are the good things you are using cannabis for? What are the

less-good things? Do you see yourself continuing to use cannabis in 1 year? 5 years? 5 years ago, did you see yourself in the situation you are in now?" These questions help to develop patients' sense of discrepancy between what they want for themselves and what their cannabis use has led to.

"I quit using cocaine, which was a much worse drug for me, but I don't want to give up marijuana." Patients who are in recovery—especially early recovery—from another substance use disorder may not want to give up using cannabis. They may see it as less problematic because the consequences of their use of other illicit drugs like heroin or cocaine were much more prominent. However, I remind them that cannabis is a mind-altering chemical that can alter their judgment and impair their ability to make good decisions. Continuing to use cannabis can lead patients back down the slippery slope of using other drugs, undoing their progress toward recovery. I tell patients that it is often easier to say no to all drug use than to determine how much drug use is too much.

Cannabis detox

Withdrawal symptoms are generally mild, but can be severe in very heavy and chronic users, with symptoms like nausea and vomiting, headache, anxiety, insomnia, and irritability. Marijuana detox is usually done in the outpatient setting, and is supportive. I tell patients that the first 5–7 days of withdrawal will be difficult, so they should not schedule any activities during that time and should concentrate on getting plenty of rest and fluids. I will sometimes prescribe an antiemetic, such as Phenergan (promethazine) or Compazine (prochlorperazine), and acetaminophen or ibuprofen for headaches.

Medications

There are no approved medications for treating cannabis use disorder. However, some people have tried dronabinol (Marinol) as substitution treatment for cannabis abuse. One clinical trial showed that it did not improve abstinence rates (Levin et al, 2011). In part, this appears to be because people who smoke are used to an immediate onset, whereas dronabinol is administered orally and its onset is delayed.

Antidepressants are helpful for longer-term depression or anxiety after immediate withdrawal. Any of the SSRIs or SNRIs are reasonable in my

⬤ **CLINICAL PEARL: Discussing Cannabis' Effects on Brain Development**

Discussing the evidence of cannabis' effects on brain development is sometimes a wake-up call for chronic cannabis users. The information tends to be of particular interest to parents of adolescents with cannabis use disorder, often encouraging their efforts to keep their children in treatment.

experience. I avoid benzodiazepines due to the potential for misuse, especially in someone who has already established a substance use disorder.

Behavioral treatment

Behavioral treatment is the mainstay of treatment for cannabis use disorder. Some patients will want to reduce their use to a controlled level instead of quitting completely; I remind them that it can be hard to determine what a safe level of use really is. If a patient is reluctant to cut down or quit, I will say, "Let's do a trial of abstinence," or, "Let's try cutting down your use for a specified period." I usually recommend a trial of abstinence for at least 1 month, ideally 3 months. I justify this to the patient by saying, "This will help us determine whether cannabis may actually be doing something beneficial." Often the patient will see an improvement in other issues with a reduction of cannabis use, which helps make the case to extend the trial.

Typical referral resources include 12-step self-help groups such as Narcotics Anonymous (NA), individual counseling with a therapist, or residential treatment if warranted by the patient's environment or severity of use. NA groups have many members who have used cannabis regularly, even if that is not their drug of choice, so patients with a primary cannabis use disorder who have not used other illicit substances can still find meaning in attending these meetings. They will also be able to find a sponsor who has experience and familiarity with the challenges they are facing. Occasionally, patients will attend an NA meeting where members do not regard cannabis as a drug of abuse. I always ask patients what they thought of their meetings, and if I hear something concerning, I will help the patient process it or recommend changing to a different meeting.

Individual therapy can help address maladaptive coping skills, or develop coping skills a patient might lack due to early age of onset of cannabis use.

CASE CONCLUSION: *I use motivational interviewing to help J recognize the connection between his cannabis use and his anxiety and inability to complete college. He agrees that reducing or eliminating his use would be worthwhile. We negotiate a controlled reduction in use as opposed to quitting cold turkey. I propose first decreasing from his usual 6 joints per day to 4 or 5 joints per day. A few weeks later, he is down to 4 joints a day, and he recognizes that this small reduction has helped him feel better overall. I continue working with him to set short-term goals, and we discuss ways for him to avoid high-risk situations. I also refer him to an individual therapist for anxiety coping skills. Eventually, J is no longer using daily, and although he has a hard time imagining himself completely abstinent, he realizes that his reduction in use has alleviated most of his anxiety. He goes back to school and does well, using cannabis only every few weeks.*

Self-Test Questions

1. A 26-year-old man gradually develops paranoia and psychosis over 8 months, until he is hospitalized for a psychotic break. He admits to smoking marijuana regularly since the age of 14. He is diagnosed with paranoid schizophrenia and started on medication. Which of the following best characterizes the current science regarding the relationship between cannabis use and psychotic disorders?
   a. Cannabis use is a risk factor for development of a psychotic disorder
   b. Development of a psychotic disorder is independent of cannabis use
   c. Prodromal schizophrenic symptoms are effectively ameliorated by cannabis
   d. Schizophrenia is caused by early initiation of cannabis

2. A 19-year-old woman has been smoking 4 cannabis joints daily for the past 10 months. She is stopped by the police for driving erratically and is held in jail over the weekend until her court hearing on Monday. While unable to use cannabis in jail, which of the following sets of symptoms is she most likely to experience?
   a. Muscle twitches, lacrimation, rhinorrhea, diarrhea
   b. Nausea, vomiting, headache, irritability
   c. Pupil dilation, hallucinations, tachycardia, hypertension
   d. Slurred speech, ataxia, hypotension, vomiting

3. A 24-year-old male began using cannabis at age 13 and escalated to daily use at age 17. He was an average student in junior high school, but his school performance and grades fell during his last years of high school because he found studying difficult and had a hard time making himself do homework or complete school projects. He thought about going to a community college, but he missed the application deadlines several times. He took a job stocking and bagging at a local grocery store because the work shifts allowed him more time to smoke cannabis at home or with his friends. Today, he is still working this job and occasionally wonders why he is not making more money. Which of the following diagnoses best describes this case?

   a. Cannabis hyperemesis syndrome
   b. Cannabis withdrawal syndrome
   c. Chronic cannabis syndrome
   d. Severe cannabis use disorder

The answer key for these self-test questions is on page 233.

Note: If you purchased CME credit with this book, your CME post-test can be accessed when you are logged in at www.thecarlatreport.com/AddictionGuide. Please keep in mind that the question and answer order for that CME post-test are different than what you see in these self-test study questions.

CHAPTER 11

Opioids

> "I'd felt the pop of the needle sliding into my veins,
> like a fang into flesh. I'd been enveloped in the
> golden haze where nothing is wrong even when
> everything is falling apart. A dance with a hypodermic
> fiend, my hands in the claws of a vulture."
> Taylor Rhodes, *Sixteenth Notes: The Breaking
> of the Rose-Colored Glasses*

TAKE HOME POINTS

- Assess the severity of the opioid problem.
- Use outpatient tapering for patients prescribed opioid analgesics for a specific pain diagnosis.
- Use intensive detox for patients with more severe addictions and those with comorbid medical or psychiatric disorders.
- Use methadone for patients with limited recovery resources, multiple previous relapses, no health insurance, or a need for close monitoring due to history of overdose or diversion.
- Use buprenorphine for patients with access to recovery resources, such as a therapist or Narcotics Anonymous groups, as well as health insurance or adequate financial support from a job or family.

CASE VIGNETTE: *F is a 23-year-old female, self-referred. She says her parents pressured her to make an appointment and are threatening to kick her out of the house because they found her stealing her father's Percocet tablets. F dropped out of college after completing her sophomore year and has been living with her parents ever since. She has had several jobs, but has been repeatedly fired for various reasons. She says her parents think* *she has a drug problem, but she disagrees. What are your initial guesses as to the extent of F's opiate problem? How would you proceed with your diagnostic assessment?*

ESSENTIALS OF OPIOIDS

First, let's clarify the terminology. What is the difference between opioid, opiates, and opium? In modern parlance, "opioid" is a comprehensive term that includes every single substance that stimulates opioid receptors in the brain. This includes both natural substances (eg, derived directly from the opium poppy, such as morphine) and synthetic substances (eg, created in a lab, such as hydrocodone). "Opiate" is often used interchangeably with opioid, though many use the word opiate specifically to refer to natural substances derived from opium—as I do in this chapter. "Opium" is the specific sticky residue that can be extracted from the opium poppy. Opium has been in use since as early as 4000 BC.

I've created a table to allow you to quickly compare any of the commonly used types of opioids (see Table 11-1). For now, here's an overview.

Morphine and codeine are natural components of the opium poppy, and both were discovered in the early 1800s. Morphine was widely used as an analgesic during the U.S. Civil War. Most subsequent opioids (including heroin, hydrocodone, oxycodone, and buprenorphine) are termed "semisynthetics," meaning they were all originally derived from one of opium's components. Finally, there are more modern opioids synthesized from basic chemicals in labs, such as methadone, fentanyl, and tramadol. Generally, synthetic opioids have been developed with higher potency or longer duration of action.

Regardless of the origin, opioids are full mu-opioid receptor agonists with very similar effects (analgesia, euphoria, sedation) and side effects (nausea, constipation, itching). Differences between these substances are due to lipid solubility (which affects the rate at which a substance crosses the blood-brain barrier to produce the main opioid effects) and metabolism (which affects a substance's duration of action).

The only illegal opioid is heroin (DEA Schedule I). Other opioids are found in schedules II, III, or IV, depending on how widespread an opioid is, its potential for abuse, and other factors. Drugs are sometimes switched to different schedules as conditions change. For example, hydrocodone was reclassified from Schedule III to Schedule II based on epidemiologic data indicating that it was more likely to be abused when less restricted, and tramadol was initially unscheduled, but after long-term post-marketing surveillance, it was placed on Schedule IV in 2015.

The popularity of heroin as a drug of abuse peaked in the 1960s, but declined somewhat during the 1970s and 1980s due to greater awareness of the risks of overdose and the increased popularity of cocaine. Throughout the 1990s and 2000s, liberal prescription of opioid analgesics for acute and chronic pain led to diversion for illicit use. Heroin use has again become a growing epidemic, because authorities have taken measures to clamp down on prescription opioid abuse, and heroin is cheaper and readily available on the streets.

Over 2 million people in the U.S. have abused prescription opioids, and the trend had been increasing throughout the 2000s, although the rate of use is starting to plateau. Around half a million people currently use heroin, but these numbers are increasing along with the numbers presenting for treatment of opioid use disorder.

> ### ⬤ CLINICAL PEARL: Side Effects to Motivate Patients
>
> *Many users don't realize that opioid use causes irregular periods or erectile dysfunction. By pointing out these effects, you can often generate more motivation to quit: "You may not realize it, but your irregular periods have a specific cause, which is your opioid use."*

Immediate effects

Psychological effects: euphoria, tranquility, and a mild sleepiness. Opioid-induced drowsiness is referred to as "the nod" because users easily nod off to sleep with their chin lowering to their chest, then startle awake—like drowsy students listening to a boring lecture.

Physical effects:

- *Digestive system.* There are opioid receptors in smooth muscle, especially in the digestive system in muscle groups that are responsible for peristalsis in the esophagus and intestines. Nausea is a common—nearly universal—side effect, though tolerance can develop. Quieting of the

TABLE 11-1. Commonly Abused Opioids

Opioid	Origin, Year	Brand Names	Street Names	Equianalgesic Doses
Buprenorphine	Semisynthetic, 1978	Subutex	Bupe	5 mg sublingual
Buprenorphine/naloxone	Semisynthetic, 2002	Suboxone, Zubsolv, Bunavail	Bupe, sobos, stop signs	Depends on product (sublingual tablet/film, buccal film)
Codeine	Opium poppy, 1832	Robitussin	Cody, robo, sizzurp, purple drank	200 mg oral
Fentanyl	Synthetic, 1960	Duragesic, Actiq, Fentora	China white, China girl, TNT	Depends on product (lozenge, buccal tablet, transdermal patch)
Heroin	Semisynthetic from morphine, 1874	illicit	H, dope, smack, horse, black tar	Wide variability due to adulteration
Hydrocodone	Semisynthetic from codeine, 1920	Vicodin, Lortab	Vikes, hykes	30 mg oral
Hydromorphone	Semisynthetic from morphine, 1924	Dilaudid	Dillies, D-lights, beans, drugstore dope	7.5 mg oral
Meperidine	Synthetic, 1939	Demerol, Mepergan	Demmies	300 mg oral
Methadone	Synthetic, 1937	Dolophine, Methadose	Meth, biscuits, fizzies	20 mg (acute), 2 mg–4 mg (chronic) oral
Morphine	Opium poppy, 1804	MSIR, MSContin		30 mg oral
Oxycodone	Semisynthetic from thebaine, 1917	Percocet, OxyContin	Oxy, OC, percs, hillbilly heroin	20 mg oral
Oxymorphone	Semisynthetic, 1914	Opana	Blue heaven, Mrs. O	10 mg oral
Tramadol	Synthetic, 1977	Ultram, Ultracet		200 mg oral

large intestine leads to constipation, which is also nearly universal among opioid users, and tolerance rarely develops for constipation.

- *Skin.* Opioids increase histamine release, which causes itching over all skin surfaces.
- *Eyes.* Opioids have a parasympathetic effect on the eyes, causing pupillary constriction (pinpoint pupils).
- *Breathing.* Respiratory depression by opioids is due to a central effect on the respiratory drive. This results in a slower breathing rate, even at low doses, and can lead to hypoxia in overdose.
- *Reproductive system.* Frequent use of opioids results in irregular menstrual cycles in women, lowered libido in both sexes, and erectile dysfunction in men due to reduction in testosterone levels.

Long-term effects

- Constipation is a long-term effect, and chronic users will typically have only a couple of bowel movements a week instead of every day. They will put up with it.
- *Reproductive system.* Opioids lower testosterone levels, resulting in decreased libido and erectile dysfunction in men. This is often treatable with sildenafil (Viagra). Women who use opioids regularly will develop irregular menstrual cycles. This results in reduced fertility, but not complete contraception. A woman may still conceive, and it may take longer for her to realize she is pregnant because she is used to missing menstrual cycles.
- *Route of administration effects.* IV use over time results in track marks, which are thin lines of callus-like skin that follow the course of a vein. This is due to repeated injection in the same vein, but moving down the course of the vein for fresh injection sites as the previous sites become scarred. IV injection of drugs carries high risk for local infections like abscesses, or more dangerous infections such as endocarditis.

Withdrawal

It takes only 2 weeks of regular use (2 or 3 times a day) to establish tolerance. Withdrawal from opioids is very much like a case of the flu, and on the street it's referred to as "the superflu" or "being dope sick." Although not life-threatening, the process is very unpleasant without a medically supervised detox protocol. The early symptoms are anxiety, craving, nausea, aches in the lower back areas and legs, muscle cramps, and possibly diarrhea. Symptoms get worse and progress to runny nose, watery eyes, intestinal cramps, vomiting, muscle twitches, and the famous "cold turkey" gooseflesh. Symptoms peak in 12 hours or so, last for 3 to 4 days, then resolve over the next few days, giving a maximum of 7 days for the withdrawal to run its course.

Although it's possible to withdraw without a detox regimen, relapse rates are high. You should instruct your patients to treat withdrawal like a bad case of the flu: with plenty of fluids, OTC cold remedies like Tylenol, antihistamines, decongestants, and loperamide for diarrhea (loperamide is an opioid, but it doesn't cross the blood-brain barrier).

Several clinical scales have been developed to measure the severity of opioid withdrawal symptoms. These include the Short Opioid Withdrawal Scale (SOWS), the Clinical Opioid Withdrawal Scale (COWS), and others.

> **FUN FACT: Origins of "Cold Turkey" and "Kicking the Habit"**
>
> "Going cold turkey" has become a colloquial term to describe abrupt withdrawal from any substance (tobacco, sugar, caffeine) or activity (like watching TV or using social media). It originally came from the piloerection seen in opioid withdrawal, a symptom that looks like the flesh of a plucked frozen turkey. The term "let's talk turkey" has a similar origin and means abruptly changing the subject to discuss something of importance.
>
> Where does the expression "kicking the habit" come from? It refers to the leg muscle twitches experienced in opioid withdrawal, which look like kicking.

The scales usually assign 1 or 2 points for each objective symptom observed by the rater. Some scales even link the severity (by number of points) to a specific dose of methadone or buprenorphine. See the COWS as an example in the Appendix.

ASSESSMENT

Returning to my patient F, the first step in the evaluation is determining how severe the problem is. Here are some guidelines for making that assessment. I view opioid use disorder as falling on a spectrum from mild to severe. These examples (of typical patients who would fall into a given category) roughly correspond to the DSM-5 criteria for opioid use disorder severity—see Chapter 1 for more on making a diagnosis with DSM-5 criteria.

Mild:

- Takes a low dose of a low-potency opioid (like codeine)
- First received opioids as a prescription for a pain issue, such as headaches
- Able to maintain a job or a relationship, and to appear normal-functioning to others

Moderate:

- Uses opioids daily or nearly daily
- Has withdrawal symptoms
- Experiences some consequences due to opioid use, such as having lost a significant relationship or even a job

- Has no opioid-related health problems
- Has not committed crimes to support a drug habit

Severe:

- Uses opioids multiple times throughout the day to avoid severe withdrawal symptoms
- Has lost relationships with people who do not use drugs
- Spends significant amounts of money on illegal opioids
- Commits crimes to support habit, usually shoplifting or petty theft
- May have switched to intranasal or IV use to overcome effects of tolerance and reduce costs
- Has a history of serious health consequences such as accidental overdose, abscesses at injection sites, or blood-borne infections such as HIV or hepatitis B or C viruses

---

CASE REVISITED: *While F presents as a well-groomed young woman who relates to me appropriately and without signs of either withdrawal or intoxication, I suspect her problem is more than just mild, because she had gone to the extreme of stealing a family member's Percocet, risking loss of housing in the process. I diagnose her with opioid use disorder, moderate. In addition, she has chronic depressive symptoms, which I diagnose as dysthymia.*

Motivational interviewing

As you begin an in-depth assessment of a patient's issues, it's important not to sound judgmental or accusatory. Opioid use disorder is a chronic condition, and you'll want to build a strong alliance with the patient in order to provide real help. I suggest beginning assessment interviews by showing interest in a general way. Ask about the patient's background: "Where are you from?" "What do you do for work and for fun?" and so on. Keep things relatively nonpsychiatric at first, and let the patient be your guide.

I often use motivational interviewing techniques during my initial evaluations (see Chapter 4 for more information). Patients are often in some degree of denial about their problem. In motivational interviewing, I acknowledge that this ambivalence is normal, and my goal is to help people to recognize that there just might be a problem here.

⬤ **DOCTOR-PATIENT DIALOGUE: Using Motivational Interviewing Techniques in Identifying the Problem**

Doctor: You said that your parents caught you taking some Percocet. Can you tell me more about what happened?

F: My dad never uses it anyway; it was for some surgery he had a year ago. I didn't think there was any harm in it.

Doctor: I get that. And did you feel you needed the Percocet more than he did?

F: I don't need it. I just thought it would be nice to have some for when I get stressed out. Unfortunately, I was stupid and did it when they were in the house. Now they think I have this huge drug problem.

Doctor: Are they worried that you use Percocet to get high?

F: Yeah, but it's not like that—I'm not an addict. I just use it to take the edge off things. But now I'm really in hot water with my parents.

Doctor: So the problem isn't that you take Percocet; the problem is that you got caught taking Percocet. You got caught because you took it when your parents were at home. Was there a reason that you couldn't wait for them to leave? [There's an opening here to explore whether the patient feels she has lost control over her cravings for the drug.]

F: No. Like I said, I was stupid. I was just feeling really stressed that day, and I saw it there and I couldn't really stop myself. I guess I was feeling weak that day.

Doctor: So it sounds like your wanting the Percocet kind of overcame your best judgment, at least for that moment.

F: I felt like I really had to have some right then. But that doesn't make me an addict!

Doctor: You don't feel like an addict at all. Is it just that sometimes you have a problem having control over your urges?

F: Maybe so.

In this snippet, F opens the door to the possibility that she does, in fact, have a problem with Percocet. Notice how we've gotten to that point. I do not say, "It's pretty clear that you have a problem with opioids if you're stealing pills from your parents." Instead, I follow her lead, reflecting her statements but also helping her to get to the point of acknowledging a problem. While this technique may seem very indirect and slow, in my experience being nonconfrontational is important and pays dividends in the degree of trust patients will develop in you.

Over time, I help patients to see the discrepancy between where they are now and where they would like to be. Then I help them understand some of the things they can work on to achieve their goals. F eventually understands that her goal is to have a good relationship with her parents, and that her addiction to Percocet is impeding that. She agrees that working toward tapering off the Percocet is a worthwhile strategy.

Common forms of denial

In asking patients about their opioid use, I have encountered many forms of denial. Here are some of the more common ones.

"My problem isn't very serious." Even people who acknowledge that they have a problem are very good at compartmentalizing—using both ambivalence and denial. They may say, "Well, I just need help with the physical part of my addiction. If I could do a quick detox, I'd be fine. I don't need to do anything else beyond that." But in fact, most patients are likely to quickly relapse without other support.

"I don't have a drug problem; I just use it sometimes to deal with stress." Self-medicating is very common. People will use what they have at hand to self-treat their depression or anxiety symptoms without recognizing it. They may use their Vicodin in the same way others would "drown their sorrows" in alcohol.

When patients acknowledge that they use opioids for emotional issues, I might respond with, "Is that giving you the kind of emotional stability you want? After all, there are other ways to get through tough days. Have you really considered the potential consequences, including your health, the potential legal issues, and how others would perceive you for doing this sort of thing?" This will often lead to a discussion of alternative treatments, like counseling or psychiatric medications.

"I have control over how much I take." People often overestimate how much control they have over their use of opioids. Things may appear relatively

stable from their point of view, but something unexpected may happen, causing more stress and a temporary escalation of use—that is, until they realize they can't cut back to what they were taking before. And if they keep increasing their dose, tolerance and withdrawal symptoms appear. Such symptoms may drive people to do more egregious things to obtain their fix, and they may start to recognize they don't want to live their lives this way.

"I'm using the drugs for physical pain; it's not an addiction." One of the main challenges is to help people acknowledge what sort of pain they are using the drugs to address—physical, emotional, or both. Patients commonly receive an opioid prescription for physical pain, then continue to use opioids for other reasons. I try to help them recognize that there's a difference between emotional pain and physical pain. The medication may temporarily alleviate some symptoms of both, but there are also negative aspects of using an opioid this way, and I help patients work through these aspects.

Questions I always ask my opioid-using patients

Here are some questions that I ask all my patients who are using opioids.

Question	Why I Ask It
How much have you been using recently?	Determine level of tolerance
How often do you need to use?	Determine level of tolerance
What has been your longest period of abstinence?	Ability to remain abstinent, predictor of potential success
Have you ever injected?	Risky behavior
How do you support your habit?	Risky behavior

Medical issues and labs

If your patient has been using heroin, or has been abusing prescription opioids by snorting or injecting, you should make sure some basic labs have been ordered, either by you or the patient's primary care doctor. These include tests for:

• HIV
• Hepatitis A, B, and C
• Complete blood count
• Liver function tests

For patients who are negative for hepatitis A and B, I recommend that they get vaccinated for both, because they are at high risk for getting exposed to the viruses in the future.

TREATMENT

There are many treatment strategies, and different patients are receptive to different approaches. The three main treatment options are:
1. Outpatient tapering
2. Detox (outpatient or inpatient)
3. Maintenance treatment

Outpatient tapering

Some patients can gradually taper down their use of oral opioids without a specific detox protocol. For the most part, these are patients who have been able to obtain the medications legitimately. For example, patients may have started taking opioids because of some dental work, but later found that they became psychologically, then physically dependent. They have been obtaining their drugs by going to multiple providers, or perhaps one provider has continued to provide refills. It would be reasonable in this context to try a therapeutic taper. In my experience, the taper will go more successfully if you taper more slowly at the beginning and at the end.

In F's case, for example, she has a habit of about 6 Percocets per day. She is not interested in an inpatient detox, nor do I think one is necessary. We therefore come up with a fairly simple tapering schedule: Reduce by half a tablet every 3 to 4 days. I reassure F that she is in control of the tapering process; she can slow down the rate if she becomes too uncomfortable from withdrawal symptoms, or taper a little faster if she wishes. I find that giving patients "permission" in this way helps them invest in the process more.

At the initial visit, I will typically order a urine drug test to verify what the patient has told me about recent use. In addition to a referral to a therapist if necessary for any comorbid disorder (such as F's dysthymia), I would recommend that the patient go to self-help groups such as Narcotics Anonymous, Secular Organization for Sobriety, or SMART Recovery (see Chapter 5 on 12-step programs and similar groups).

CASE REVISITED: *When F returns for her next appointment, she says she was able to taper from 6 to 4 Percocets per day, and although she has been* *experiencing transient insomnia and anxiety, she is willing to continue with the plan. I recommend slowing the taper down a bit to avoid these symptoms.*

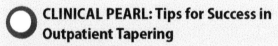

CLINICAL PEARL: Tips for Success in Outpatient Tapering

Tapering down opioids can be difficult. Here are some tips:
– Slow down the taper
– Switch to a different opioid for the taper
– Reassure patients that they are in control of the tapering process

Tapering by switching to a different opioid

Another option is to switch your patient to a different, usually long-acting, opioid before doing the taper, often either buprenorphine or methadone (see sections below for details on these agents). One reason to do this is to interrupt the positive associations a patient might have made with a particular drug. In addition, switching to a longer-acting drug makes for less frequent dosing. The fewer points during the day that people have to choose between taking or not taking something, the more successful they'll be in following a tapering schedule.

Outpatient detox

Detox (detoxification), at its core, is a more medically supervised version of tapering. It's usually reserved for those with more severe problems.

My approach to outpatient detox is similar to the outpatient tapering protocol I've outlined with F, except that I'll ask the patient to return for more frequent appointments, and I will make referrals to more resources, such as an intensive outpatient program. I will almost always switch the patient to a longer-acting opioid, either methadone or buprenorphine—this is less common in outpatient tapering. In addition, I may offer extra "comfort" medications to address the common detox symptoms of opioid withdrawal (see Table 11-2).

For inpatient detox, the same medication strategy applies, except that everything occurs in an inpatient environment with intensive monitoring for withdrawal symptoms. Patients will also get individual and group

TABLE 11-2. Medications Useful for Opioid Withdrawal Symptoms

Withdrawal Symptom	Medication	Typical Dosing/Notes
Multiple general symptoms	clonidine	0.1 mg–0.2 mg PO every 6 hours, or 0.3 mg transdermal patch (patient leaves single patch on skin for 7 days)
Nausea	prochlorperazine	5 mg–10 mg PO every 6 hours PRN
Diarrhea	loperamide	2 mg, 1–2 tablets PO every 6 hours PRN
Aches	ibuprofen	200 mg, 1–2 tablets PO every 8 hours PRN
Insomnia	trazodone	50 mg PO at bedtime

psychotherapy, as well as 12-step meetings, when the detox occurs at an addiction treatment program facility; they are usually better able to participate after the initial few days of detox. This extra support is not usually available right away in a hospital's medical or psychiatric inpatient unit.

Relapse rates are high even with a detox regimen, but patients who quit cold turkey often don't make it through withdrawal before relapsing. Contrary to popular belief, people can die from unsupervised opioid withdrawal, particularly if they have underlying conditions like diabetes or cardiac arrhythmia that may be worsened by electrolyte imbalances caused by nausea and vomiting.

Buprenorphine treatment

Buprenorphine is a semisynthetic opioid that has been available as an analgesic since 1981. It has long been used to treat acute pain and comes in different forms, including injectable, sublingual, and transdermal patch.

How did buprenorphine end up playing such a central role in treating opioid abuse? Unlike other opioid products such as codeine, hydrocodone, oxycodone, methadone, and even heroin, buprenorphine is a partial agonist—in other words, a combined opioid agonist/antagonist. This means it occupies the opioid receptors, but doesn't cause quite the same intensity of receptor activation (or "high") as full opioid agonists. This is an advantage for people who are in treatment, because it gives them enough of an effect to ward off withdrawal, but doesn't make them so high that they are reminded of—and tempted by—the high from other opioids. The bottom line is that buprenorphine, with its push/pull agonist/antagonist properties, is less likely to be abused than its opioid cousins. This in itself makes it a good choice for maintenance treatment, but buprenorphine is also much less likely to produce respiratory arrest in overdose.

The buprenorphine mono product (brand name Subutex) has been generic for a few years and is relatively cheap; some insurance companies have it on their preferred formulary list. For many addiction specialists, plain old buprenorphine is the treatment of choice for both detox and opioid maintenance.

Buprenorphine is a Schedule III controlled substance, so it's less restricted than methadone (which is Schedule II). Patients can get a 1-month prescription from a buprenorphine provider with up to 5 refills—although monthly visits at minimum are generally recommended. One of the reasons buprenorphine is less restricted is its safety profile—as an opioid agonist/antagonist, it's more difficult to overdose on buprenorphine than it is on methadone. But there's a catch: To prescribe buprenorphine (with or without naloxone; see below), you need a waiver from the Department of Health and Human Services—a system that was established as part of the Drug Addiction Treatment Act of 2000. You must complete an 8-hour training to obtain this waiver, which will then enable you to prescribe buprenorphine to as many as 100 patients. The Comprehensive Addiction Recovery Act of 2016 raised the patient limit to 275 for addiction treatment providers with advanced training.

Buprenorphine/naloxone

Given that buprenorphine alone is an effective treatment for opioid addiction, why did drug makers create a combination pill of buprenorphine and naloxone? Wouldn't naloxone—an opioid blocker used to reverse opioid overdoses—neutralize buprenorphine's effectiveness, rendering it useless? Not if the pill is taken sublingually, as directed. When buprenorphine is absorbed through the mouth's mucosal lining, it works fine—but naloxone is then inactivated. However, if the pill is ground up and dissolved for injection, the naloxone is very much active and will prevent the user from getting high. So naloxone was added to reduce the potential for abuse by injection.

How to start patients on buprenorphine: Induction

CASE VIGNETTE: *A is a 24-year-old man who presents for outpatient opioid detox. He began using extended-release oxycodone (OxyContin)* *during his freshman year of college, which he has always bought illegally. He has snorted heroin a few times, but has not injected any drugs. He has experienced many consequences of his opioid use, including guilt about lying to friends and family, debt from buying illegal drugs, loss of a girlfriend, significant depression, and opioid withdrawal symptoms. He is ready to get off opioid analgesics, but is not interested in residential addiction treatment because of his work schedule. However, he can take a day off work to come in for a buprenorphine induction.*

Induction refers to the somewhat complicated process of starting an opioid-dependent patient on buprenorphine (by "buprenorphine" I am referring to any of the preparations, whether mono or combined with naloxone). It can be done in an outpatient setting, and depending on the ultimate dose (based on a patient's tolerance), the process can take 1–2 days.

I start by emphasizing to patients that they should not use opioids for about 24 hours before presenting for induction—otherwise the first dose will cause an unpleasant withdrawal experience. Buprenorphine treatment should be started in the early stage of withdrawal, which generally means that patients will have noticed some nausea and muscle achiness, rated at 2 or 3 points on the COWS (see Appendix). Your starting dose of buprenorphine will be 2 mg–4 mg, repeated every hour or two until patients are comfortable.

Most forms of buprenorphine are administered sublingually. The tablets should not be swallowed; buprenorphine has poor oral bioavailability, so a swallowed tablet is a waste of money for the patient. They take at least 5 minutes to dissolve, longer if more than one is needed per dose. I tell patients to rinse their mouth out thoroughly, and then to get it nice and moist. I then have patients place 1 or 2 tablets (or films) under the tongue and allow several minutes for the dose to dissolve completely. Patients should not talk or swallow while the medication is dissolving; I try to only ask yes-or-no questions until the medication is gone. It is fine to drink something immediately after the dose has dissolved, which can help with the medicinal taste.

I check on patients every hour or so throughout the induction, which usually lasts 4–8 hours. Our clinic has a comfortable waiting room with Wi-Fi, a DVD player, and magazines; I tell patients, "You're going to be hanging out for a while. There's a bathroom very close by." Medical

— BUPRENORPHINE INDUCTION CHEAT SHEET —

1. Patient must be in early withdrawal
2. Buprenorphine, 2 mg–4 mg sublingually every hour or two while in office
3. At end of induction, friend drives patient home
4. Day 2: Give entire day 1 dose at once in office
5. Add doses if needed
6. Once dose is finalized, make follow-up appointment for 1 week or less

personnel, myself or my nurse, check on them regularly, and they can get someone's attention right away.

After the second dose, most people feel much better physically, so then it's just a matter of titrating up to where they feel comfortable without being too sedated. Depending on their tolerance, typical maintenance doses range from about 10 mg to 20 mg a day.

At the end of the first day of induction, I make sure patients have someone who can drive them home. I will usually give them a prescription to pick up a small amount of buprenorphine at the pharmacy. The next morning, they come back, and we pick up where we left off the day before. I give them the whole first day's dose all at once to start with and make sure they can tolerate it, and then if necessary go up from there. It usually takes us two days to find the right dose; in cases where it takes longer, I'll have the patient come into the office for a few more days.

CASE CONCLUSION: *A arrives at the clinic at 8:30 a.m. to start the induction process. He says he has not used any opioids for 2 days since his initial visit. As a result, he is experiencing opioid withdrawal symptoms: nausea, diarrhea, and cravings. I give A an initial dose of 4 mg of Suboxone (buprenorphine/naloxone). An hour later, he still has significant withdrawal symptoms, so I give him another 4 mg. About an hour later, he reports 80% improvement in his symptoms, and I give him a 2 mg dose. The next time I check on him, A's withdrawal symptoms have completely subsided, and he denies any opioid side effects such as sedation. His mother drives him home.*

A comes back the next morning feeling well. He reports no withdrawal symptoms overnight and denies using any extra opioids or other drugs. I have him take the total dose he had taken the day before all at once: 10 mg of Suboxone. He is monitored for 90 minutes with no problems. I write him a prescription for 4 days' worth of Suboxone, enough to last until his next follow-up appointment. I also encourage A to go to local Narcotics Anonymous meetings and find a therapist.

After the induction, I will generally see patients weekly, which allows me to make dosage adjustments as needed. I will increase the dose if there are still cravings and withdrawal symptoms, or reduce it if there are opioid side effects, such as constipation or oversedation.

While it's not always easy to determine the right amount of buprenorphine for a given patient, it's important to do your best. Some patients may exaggerate their withdrawal symptoms to obtain higher doses of buprenorphine, and then divert the extra pills to the black market, either for profit or in exchange for other drugs that the patient likes better. This is a good reason to do regular random urine drug testing (see Chapter 2) not only for illicit drugs, but also for the presence of buprenorphine (or its metabolite, norbuprenorphine). It is harder to detect diversion if the patient is taking some and selling some, although establishing a good rapport with the patient can reduce the chances of being fooled. Another way to detect diversion is with random short-notice medication counts (have patients bring in all their leftover medication between visits on short notice—less than 24 hours—to establish whether they are using it at the expected rate), but this takes time, so I only do it for patients I'm especially concerned about.

Buprenorphine maintenance vs. tapering

Once we have arrived at a stable dose of buprenorphine, I talk with patients about how long they will need to stay on it. Some people need more time on the medication—months to years—because of the severity of their addiction and the harsh consequences of relapse. Having such patients on a maintenance dose for many months allows them time to work on the behavioral components that they are learning in therapy or in 12-step programs. Other patients may start from a better place—a less severe usage problem and a good support system. These patients might be ready for a taper fairly soon after starting on buprenorphine.

In any case, once everyone involved in the patient's treatment—including the patient—recognizes that some stability has been achieved, we talk about decreasing the dose. The taper is fairly straightforward. The smallest dosage strength is 2 mg, and patients can cut pills or strips in half and taper down in 1 mg increments. I'll have patients decrease the dose anywhere from every few days to every few weeks, depending on the time available and the patient's physical and psychological comfort level. A typical out-patient taper will take around 2 months, and this time can be lengthened depending on the patient's readiness and starting dose.

Typical causes of buprenorphine treatment failure

• Lack of support. A home environment that doesn't provide the needed support is a major cause of problems with remaining abstinent. Patients need to have family or close nonusing friends for encouragement and to help them deal with the emotional and physical ups and downs of early recovery.
• Using other drugs. Some people don't want to give up their marijuana or alcohol, which is another reason for relapse. I do random drug testing, and I let people know that their goal is going to be abstinence from all problem substances.

How to choose among the different formulations of buprenorphine

Suboxone was the first buprenorphine/naloxone product to be approved (in 2002), and in 2010 its period of marketing exclusivity expired. Since then, several versions have been introduced, and at the time of this writing there are six versions to choose from. The main factor influencing the choice of formulation tends to be the patient's insurance policy. Some insurance simply covers the cheapest formulation: the generic mono product, buprenorphine without naloxone. However, there are other more meaningful factors distinguishing the products.

Bioavailability: Bioavailability refers to the fraction of the drug that makes its way into the bloodstream and to the brain. When taken orally, typical drug molecules are absorbed by the small intestine and then delivered by portal blood vessels to the liver, which metabolizes some fraction of the drug, removing it from circulation. This is called the first-pass effect, and the degree to which it occurs varies from drug to drug. The only way to completely avoid the first-pass effect is to administer drugs intravenously, which gets 100% of the drug into systemic circulation (100% bioavailability). Another way to bypass the liver is with sublingual drugs, which dissolve under the tongue and get absorbed into the oral mucosa. These capillaries go directly to systemic circulation. Most buprenorphine/naloxone preparations exploit the oral mucosa route in some way or another, but they vary in effectiveness. The greater the bioavailability, the lower the dose required, which is why, for example, Bunavail (the citrus-flavored buccal film approved in June 2014) 4.2 mg is equivalent to sublingual bup/nal 8 mg.

Speed of onset: While all the formulations dissolve and get absorbed somewhere in the mouth, some get absorbed more quickly than others. A faster absorption means that a withdrawal patient in your office will get somewhat faster relief from those symptoms—but we're only talking about 10 or 15 minutes' difference at most.

Dose required: The more bioavailable formulations require a lower number of milligrams to achieve the same effect. A possible disadvantage is a psychological one—for example, patients who are used to taking 8 mg of Suboxone may believe they are getting too little if they are switched to a 4.2 mg equivalent dose of Bunavail. This "nocebo" effect (the opposite of the placebo effect) can be significant when it comes to subjective perceptions of opioid effects.

With all this in mind, let's go through the various formulations of buprenorphine (see Table 11-3).

In general, I favor the combination product (buprenorphine/naloxone) over the mono product because it tends to be more available in pharmacies. Some patients and their families request the combination because of naloxone's potential to help prevent abuse. There is one clear role for the mono product over the combination product: for pregnant women to reduce fetal exposure to medications, including naloxone. Recent research has shown that buprenorphine is safe and effective in pregnancy, with similar effectiveness to methadone (Jones et al, 2010; Jones et al, 2005).

Among the combination formulations, Suboxone has been around the longest and patients are most familiar with it. The strips tend to be more easily dissolvable than the sublingual Zubsolv tablets. A more recent alternative is Bunavail, a buccal patch (dissolving on the inside of the cheek as opposed to under the tongue). Its theoretical advantages are that it dissolves the fastest and allows patients to talk and eat with the patch in their mouths.

Probuphine, approved in May 2016, is an implantable version of buprenorphine that releases a consistent daily dose for 24 weeks. It uses 4

TABLE 11-3. Formulations of Buprenorphine

Generic Name (Brand Name) Year FDA Approved (Rx status) [G] denotes generic availability	Formulation and Available Strengths (mg)	Usual Dosage Range (mg)	Advantages/Disadvantages
Buprenorphine (formerly Subutex) [G] 2002	Sublingual tablets: 2, 8	4–24 QD	*Advantages:* Original mono version; long track record; very inexpensive. Many experts find it to be just as effective as agents that include naloxone. *Disadvantage:* Since it does not contain naloxone, it can be ground up and injected.
Buprenorphine and naloxone [G] 2002 (C-III)	Sublingual tablets: bup 2/nal 0.5, 8/2	4–24 QD	*Advantages:* First combination buprenorphine/naloxone agent. Long track record; inexpensive. *Disadvantage:* Some complain about the taste.
Buprenorphine and naloxone (Suboxone) [G] 2010	Sublingual strips: bup 2/nal 0.5, 4/1, 8/2, 12/3	4–24 QD	*Advantages:* Faster absorption than tablets; easy to taper gradually because film can be cut into small sizes; packaging makes it more difficult for kids to open. *Disadvantages:* More diversion potential because strips can be easily mailed; relatively high cost.
Buprenorphine and naloxone (Bunavail) 2014 (C-III)	Buccal film: bup 2.1/nal 0.3, 4.2/0.7, 6.3/1	2.1–12.6 QD	*Advantages:* High bioavailability; fast absorption; less constipation; more convenient than other preparations because it sticks to the cheek while dissolving, allowing patients to talk. *Disadvantages:* Very high cost; may be more difficult to cut than Suboxone film, because cutting may decrease its sticking ability to cheek mucosa.
Buprenorphine and naloxone (Zubsolv) 2013 (C-III)	Sublingual tablets: bup 1.4/nal 0.36, 2.9/0.71, 5.7/1.4, 8.6/2.1, 11.4/2.9	2.9–17.2 QD	*Advantages:* Menthol flavor; higher bioavailability than generics. *Disadvantage:* Higher cost than generics.
Probuphine 2016 (C-III)	Rods implanted subdermally in the upper arm; each rod contains 74.2 mg of buprenorphine	Rods release the equivalent of 320 mg of buprenorphine over 6 months	*Advantages:* Very long-acting; consistent dosing; good bioavailability. *Disadvantages:* Requires surgical implantation; may lead to scarring; only for stable patients maintained on buprenorphine 8 mg/day or lower.

rods that must be inserted surgically in the upper arm under local anesthesia; the old rods are removed when new ones are implanted. Probuphine is for long-term maintenance in patients who are stable on buprenorphine at a maintenance dose of no more than 8 mg per day.

Methadone maintenance treatment

While any physician can prescribe methadone for pain, when used for opioid addiction, it can only be prescribed at federally licensed treatment programs—otherwise known as "methadone clinics." Patients must show up every day to receive their dose, and they must attend individual counseling sessions at least twice per month, or go to weekly group sessions.

Why would you refer a patient to methadone maintenance over a far less restrictive buprenorphine maintenance program? Generally, the best candidates for methadone maintenance are those who need the extra supervision of daily monitoring. These include patients who have had multiple accidental overdoses, those who have diverted their meds, and those with severe psychiatric or medical problems. Another advantage of methadone maintenance is that the clinics are often publicly funded, so poorer patients will pay less out of pocket.

⊘ METHADONE—AT A GLANCE	
Indications	Pain, opioid addiction
Dosages available	5 mg tablets, 10 mg tablets, 40 mg dispersible tablets, liquid elixir 1 mg/ml
Target dosages	80 mg–120 mg/day
Special considerations	When used for opioid addiction, can be given only in approved treatment program

In terms of pharmacology, methadone is the better choice for patients who have very high tolerance to opioids. High tolerance is the result of using high amounts daily, especially heroin of high purity (sometimes called a "dealer's habit"). Buprenorphine often won't work for these patients because its agonist-antagonist effects mean that higher doses (over 32 mg per day) can cause paradoxical symptoms of opioid withdrawal and anxiety. With methadone, on the other hand, there is no ceiling effect, and the dose can be raised as high as needed to prevent withdrawal symptoms and cravings.

> ## CAUTION! Methadone for Detox
>
> ⚠️ Methadone is a particularly long-acting opioid. Patients may not notice the effects as quickly as they are used to, and might be tempted to take extra doses initially. These doses can catch up to them all at once, and patients may accidentally overdose. Don't prescribe methadone for detox unless you have experience managing opioid withdrawal.

Of course, the lack of a ceiling dose also leads to a big disadvantage of methadone: It has a greater potential for lethal overdose compared to buprenorphine. This is one reason methadone maintenance treatment has closer monitoring. Another disadvantage of methadone is that there are more drug interactions that can affect its level. Methadone is metabolized mainly by CYP 3A4. Risperidone, rifampicin, and many antiretroviral medications can lower serum methadone levels, resulting in opioid withdrawal symptoms. Conversely, diazepam, fluoxetine, and erythromycin can elevate methadone levels, increasing the risk of overdose. Finally, although rare, methadone use has been associated with cardiac QTc interval prolongation, which in turn can lead to torsades de pointes, a potentially fatal arrhythmia.

Despite the disadvantages of methadone, in my clinical experience, the treatment is worth it for patients with severe opioid use disorder. Such patients have a very high mortality risk if they are not in treatment and are injecting high doses of illicit drugs.

How to dose methadone

Choosing the initial dose of methadone maintenance treatment is both art and science, dependent on how much and how frequently the patient has been using. The higher a patient's use, the higher the starting dose that should be given to avoid withdrawal. A typical initial dose is 20 mg–30 mg, usually given as a liquid and often diluted with juice or artificially colored water. Each client receives a full cup of uniformly colored liquid regardless of the dose of methadone, in order to reduce anxiety among clients about differences in dose. The dilution also reduces the likelihood of a patient injecting "take home" doses of methadone (more on this shortly); the amount of liquid renders injection impractical.

The dose is titrated up over the first few days by 10 mg–20 mg each day, up to an initial target range of 60 mg–80 mg daily, with more gradual increases as needed. The dose can be fine-tuned over the first few weeks based on patient assessment and feedback. Most patients end up doing best on doses between 80 mg–120 mg per day, which is usually enough to block a euphoric high if patients choose to use illicit opioids outside of treatment.

Though we think of methadone as being given daily under supervision, some patients earn eligibility for "take home" doses. They generally need 90 days of continuous abstinence from illicit drugs (based on urine tox screens) to gain this privilege. Initial take-home doses are for 2 days at a time, usually over weekends. Clients can work their way up to getting 28 days of take-home doses at a time. At that point, clients only come to the methadone maintenance clinic once every four weeks, and periodically for group sessions or meetings with their counselor.

Another treatment for opioid use disorder: Vivitrol

🔍 VIVITROL—AT A GLANCE	
Indications	Opioid addiction, alcohol addiction
Dosages available	380 mg IM
Target dosages	380 mg IM every 4 weeks
Special considerations	Patient must have abstained from opioids for 1 week before use

Vivitrol is a long-acting injectable form of naltrexone, which is an opioid receptor blocker like naloxone. If patients try to use an opioid within four weeks of a Vivitrol injection, they won't feel a high. Thus, Vivitrol is neither a tapering tool nor an agonist maintenance medication. It is only helpful for patients who have discontinued opioids completely and are highly motivated to continue abstinence (antagonist maintenance).

Before an injection with Vivitrol, people must abstain from opioids for at least several days, preferably about a week. You may have to do a detox with methadone or buprenorphine to get patients off their preferred opioids, and then have them remain off all opioids for a few days. The injections are deep gluteal intramuscular injections performed every 4 weeks at the physician's office (the manufacturer sends the injection kits there). No special licensing is needed to administer them.

Who's most appropriate for Vivitrol? In my experience, it's patients who have a supportive home environment and access to outpatient counseling or Narcotics Anonymous meetings (or similar self-help groups). Vivitrol can be worthwhile for patients who have completed detox successfully, either inpatient or outpatient. It's also a good fit for patients who can't risk having any opioids in their systems. This includes patients who would be out of a job immediately if they failed a workplace urine test, as well as those who can't be sedated while at work due to being in a high-risk occupation (eg, health care workers, long-distance drivers, heavy machinery operators, etc).

Vivitrol is effective to extinguish use, but people may not show up for subsequent injections. Because it's not an agonist, it's also not as rewarding. In a psychiatric setting, giving someone who has a dual diagnosis an injection can give both the provider and the patient some peace of mind for a while, so that can be a part of discharge planning. A potential danger with Vivitrol is that if patients decide to stop getting the injection so that they can start using again, they will have lost some of their opioid tolerance, and the amount of heroin that once made them high could easily cause an overdose. This is something you may want to warn some patients about.

Preventing disaster: Using naloxone

🔍 NALOXONE—AT A GLANCE	
Indication	Opioid overdose, emergency treatment
Dosages available	4 mg/0.1 ml nasal spray; 0.4 mg/0.4 ml auto-injector
Target dosages	One spray per nostril; 0.4 mg SC or IM
Special considerations	Patient may awaken in withdrawal and agitated

Opioid overdose is treated with naloxone (Narcan). In the past, the only route of administration was intravenous, and it was used only by EMTs, police, and other first responders. Now, there is also an intranasal version of naloxone. Narcan can be administered by friends or family members instead of having to wait for emergency responders, which can be lifesaving. Often, you will be prescribing Narcan to your opioid-using patients; they will likely be in a position to rescue other users, or they will make it available to their associates for their own rescue.

When you talk to patients or bystanders about Narcan, I recommend giving them the following instructions:
• Learn how to recognize the signs of opioid overdose
• First try to awaken the patient (in case it is not an overdose)

- Give naloxone according to the package directions (many kits or pharmacies have a demonstrator kit)
- After the patient responds to the naloxone, call 911

Naloxone buys time for paramedics to arrive after an overdose. It is not complete treatment—only the first step in saving the life of an overdose victim. The person who overdosed may lapse back into unconsciousness 20 minutes after receiving naloxone when it wears off before the opioid does, so paramedics need to take the patient to the emergency department for ongoing treatment of the overdose.

Psychosocial interventions

In addition to prescribing medication, I make sure my patients are engaged in psychosocial intervention. This might be individual counseling, a group program, or involvement with a 12-step group. I want them to be working on relapse prevention, coping, and refusal skills. In their home environment, I encourage patients to rally as much support as possible from family and friends who are not using drugs.

Psychiatric medications for other symptoms

Antidepressants and other medications for anxiety can be helpful in supporting recovery, and just about any of the SSRIs and SNRIs are appropriate. Gabapentin and hydroxyzine are effective antianxiety medications that are not controlled substances. For insomnia, there are medications like trazodone or ramelteon.

Benzodiazepines are not ideal for patients in opioid recovery. They can produce a high that may lead to craving and relapse, and while it's hard to overdose on buprenorphine alone, the combination of buprenorphine and benzodiazepines can lead to fatal overdose. It's important to let patients know about this risk.

CASE CONCLUSION: *F is able to complete her taper using methadone to get completely off of opioids. She found that a long-acting opioid was easier to taper with than "playing catch-up" with short-acting Vicodin. She begins seeing a therapist for individual counseling for her dysthymia; that therapist also provides relapse prevention counseling. F tries going to a few Narcotics Anonymous meetings, and to her surprise, she finds them beneficial. She has been in recovery for two years.*

Self-Test Questions

1. A 37-year-old man comes for evaluation because of stomach cramps, diarrhea, and severe craving for opioids; these symptoms began 3 days ago when he stopped using oxycodone cold turkey after his wife threatened to leave him if he didn't quit. He has been using oxycodone daily for 15 months, but reports that 4 months ago, he rapidly escalated his daily dose to greater than 100 mg. He recently lost his job because he would leave the office to buy and use oxycodone. He has unsuccessfully tried to reduce his opioid use several times over the past 3 months. Which of the following best describes this patient's opioid use pattern?
   a. Episodic binge opioid use
   b. Opioid use disorder, moderate
   c. Opioid use disorder, severe
   d. Opioid-induced depression

2. A 22-year-old man presents requesting treatment for addiction to prescription opioid analgesics. On a daily basis, he has been using 10–12 tablets of hydrocodone with acetaminophen, which he buys illegally. He has gone to Narcotics Anonymous meetings, but would stay clean for only a day or two before relapsing due to opioid withdrawal symptoms. Which of the following treatments is most likely to help this patient stay abstinent?
   a. Acamprosate
   b. Buprenorphine with naloxone
   c. Probuphine
   d. Naloxone rescue kit

3. A 29-year-old woman has been injecting heroin for nearly 10 years. She has also sold or misused opioid analgesics prescribed to her, and has had several accidental overdoses. She has gone to a number of treatment centers for detoxification, but each time relapsed within 3 months of discharge. Because of this history, her physician would like her to be monitored on a daily basis when she takes medication for treatment of her opioid use disorder. Which of the following is the best treatment option for this patient?
   a. Methadone
   b. Buprenorphine
   c. Naloxone
   d. Probuphine

The answer key for these self-test questions is on page 233.

Note: If you purchased CME credit with this book, your CME post-test can be accessed when you are logged in at www.thecarlatreport.com/AddictionGuide. Please keep in mind that the question and answer order for that CME post-test are different than what you see in these self-test study questions.

CHAPTER 12

Stimulants

"Cocaine is God's way of saying you're making too much money."
Robin Williams

TAKE HOME POINTS

- The major stimulants of abuse are cocaine and amphetamines.
- Stimulants cause euphoria and enhanced attention, followed by a crash.
- Stimulant withdrawal causes fatigue, irritability, depression, craving, and increased appetite.
- There is no pharmacological treatment for stimulant use disorder.
- An effective behavioral treatment is contingency management.

CASE VIGNETTE: *N is a 35-year-old woman who presents to me with the chief complaint of "I have issues with cocaine." Although she referred herself to me, she was strongly encouraged to make the appointment by her boyfriend. In the past, he and N had used cocaine together, but he had dramatically reduced his use to focus on his job and their preteen son. He is unhappy with N's continued use, both because she is using his money to buy the drugs and because when she runs out of money, she gets cocaine from "friends"—he suspects she is trading sexual favors to do so.*

STIMULANT ESSENTIALS

In this chapter, we will focus on the stimulants cocaine and amphetamines (see Table 12-1) and briefly cover caffeine. Other stimulants include designer drugs such as cathinones, amphetamine derivatives including

185

TABLE 12-1. Stimulants of Abuse

Name	Brand Name	Slang Names
Cocaine	Roxane	Blow, coke, crack, lady, rock, snow
Dextroamphetamine	Adderall	Addy, smarties, uppers
Methamphetamine	Desoxyn	Black beauties, crank, crystal meth, dexies, ice, speed, uppers
Methylphenidate	Ritalin, Concerta	Rits, smart pills, vitamin R

MDMA (ecstasy), and other similar substances (see Chapter 13). Stimulants vary in their chemical structure, but they are all "sympathomimetics," meaning that they mimic the actions of the sympathetic (fight or flight) nervous system. These include the physiological changes that prepare an organism for rapid action, such as increased heart rate and blood pressure, pupillary dilation, and decreased appetite. Unfortunately, there is both a psychological and physiological crash after the effects of stimulants wear off, and the crash leads to most of the negative effects, including cravings and depression.

Overview of stimulants

Cocaine

Cocaine is a psychoactive compound that is derived from the leaves of the coca plant. Chewing coca leaves has been a part of South American culture for millennia, historically done to overcome fatigue, hunger, and thirst.

> **FUN FACT: Walking a Cocada**
>
> In South America, a "cocada" was used as a measure of distance, defined as how far a man could walk in a day while chewing coca leaves. Villages were said to be a certain number of cocadas apart.

Cocaine is rendered by placing the leaves in various solvents to produce cocaine hydrochloride, which is purified to a white powder. This powder can then be snorted, or injected when dissolved in water. Another commonly used version of cocaine is called crack. Crack is created by mixing cocaine hydrochloride powder with baking soda (to create the "freebase" form), microwaving it to make it hard, then breaking it into small chunks called rocks. This process removes the hydrochloride and lowers the substance's melting point, allowing the crack to be smoked. Smoking creates a quicker and more intense high than snorting.

In the U.S., cocaine became popular among the wealthy in the 1970s, but late in that decade, Colombian drug cartels developed crack as a less expensive alternative to cocaine powder. A rock of crack could be purchased for $10, and since it was smoked, it was easier to consume and titrate to the desired effect.

> ### NOT-SO-FUN FACT: Crack and the Open Flame
>
> Since cocaine is expensive, users don't keep it lit like a tobacco pipe; rather, they only heat it when they're ready to inhale a hit, so they are periodically applying a flame from a cigarette lighter or gas stove to the crack pipe. This can result in burns to the hands or face. Because of the impurities in crack, users can inhale soot that is vaporized along with the cocaine, which can burn the mouth or the back of the throat. Often a filter is used, which can be a piece of cloth, a fine wire mesh, or anything that will serve as a strainer. Unfortunately, the burst of hot air that comes out of the pipe can blow the filter into the back of the throat. I had a patient who accidentally inhaled the steel wool filter she used for her crack pipe; the hot metal caused her throat to swell up, requiring endotracheal intubation to allow her to breathe. What surprised me is that she did this more than once, endangering her life and ending up in the ICU twice. The famous comedian Richard Pryor suffered a severe burn injury in 1980 related to smoking crack.

Methamphetamine

Methamphetamine is simply the amphetamine molecule with a methyl group attached to allow for easier entry to the brain via the blood-brain barrier. Its effects are similar to cocaine but longer lasting (4–8 hours, as opposed to about 30 minutes for cocaine). Amphetamines block dopamine reuptake and are MAO inhibitors, enhancing the actions of the catecholamines, epinephrine and norepinephrine.

ADHD stimulants

Stimulants approved for treating ADHD are also drugs of abuse. While amphetamines (Adderall and others) and methylphenidate (Ritalin) are both addictive, Adderall has emerged as a favorite and is especially popular with younger people. Among high school and college students, Adderall and other stimulants are viewed as "smart pills," though they don't improve mastery or memory. The drugs enable students to stay awake longer to cram before exams, but most users report that taking them doesn't improve their grades.

Caffeine and energy drinks

Caffeine is different from stimulants, since it works on adenosine receptors as opposed to dopamine and is therefore not as potent. While caffeine is not problematic for most users, a subset will use larger amounts and go through a cycle of heightened energy and attention followed by withdrawal, which includes symptoms such as tiredness, headache, and irritability. In substance users, caffeine withdrawal may increase the risk of relapse to other drugs. Consuming energy drinks such as Red Bull and Monster increases the risk of caffeine problems.

Because caffeine can be a source of irritability and contribute to anxiety, reducing caffeine consumption is a relatively easy fix to improve people's moods. I'll suggest things like having smaller cups, mixing half caffeinated and half decaffeinated, or substituting other beverages like water as ways to start cutting down on coffee, tea, or soda consumption.

When assessing caffeine use, I ask patients, "How many cups of coffee do you have a day? How many cups of tea or sweet tea? How many sodas? How often do you have energy drinks?" If patients report that they use caffeine to counteract tiredness or "to get going" in the morning, I'll advise them to exercise to increase their energy level. I'll also teach them about basic sleep hygiene tips, and remind them that they'll sleep better if they don't have caffeine after dinner. Although people may say they can fall asleep fine after drinking a cup of coffee, the sleep they get is more likely to be the non-restorative type. Many people don't know caffeine has two effects on sleep: an awakening effect early on, and a sleep-depressing effect up to 12 hours later. This means if they drink coffee at 3 p.m., it could still be keeping them awake at 3 a.m. Patients will sometimes cut down on their afternoon or evening caffeine after this is explained to them.

Immediate effects

Both cocaine and meth lead to an immediate rush of euphoria, energy, and enhanced concentration. At high doses, the drugs lead to such heightened alertness that it borders on paranoia. Regular use can cause psychotic features, including auditory hallucinations and delusions of thought insertion or extraction. Although these symptoms can be clinically indistinguishable from schizophrenia, they usually subside when the drug wears off.

Cocaine and other stimulants can also cause various perceptual effects. For example, "snow lights" are flashes and colors in the periphery of a user's vision, and "coke bugs" (or "crank bugs") are a tactile hallucination of bugs crawling on the skin. The sensation caused by coke bugs is also known clinically as formication (the word is derived from the formic acid excreted by ants in the subfamily *Formicinae*). The skin lesions seen in cocaine and meth users are partially caused by this hallucination, since people will scratch and pick at their skin to get at the imagined bugs.

Heavy stimulant users often use sedatives to take the edge off the stimulant effects. Sometimes they will combine opioids with stimulants (speedballs), either by combining cocaine and heroin into one needle, or more commonly by smoking crack and snorting heroin.

Combining alcohol with cocaine also takes the edge off, but it has another popular effect: It prolongs the cocaine high. When alcohol and cocaine coexist in the bloodstream, the liver combines them to create an active metabolite called cocaethylene. Because about 40% of cocaethylene is metabolized back into cocaine, the combination effectively lengthens cocaine's half-life.

 SAD FACT: Famous Victims of Speedball Overdoses

John Belushi, 33, comedian (cocaine and heroin); died 1982

River Phoenix, 23, actor (cocaine and heroin); died 1993

Chris Farley, 33, comedian (cocaine and morphine); died 1997

Philip Seymour Hoffman, 46, actor (cocaine, heroin, benzodiazepines, and amphetamines); died 2014

Unlike drugs such as sedatives and opioids, people don't use stimulants at a constant level; instead, they use intensely for a short period of time, called a run or spree. This can last for several hours or several days, sometimes ending only when users run out of money, drug, or dopamine. Then they crash, and after a period of not wanting to use, they start to have cravings.

Long-term effects

Psychiatric syndromes, such as depression and psychosis, can persist between periods of stimulant use.

A Parkinson-like syndrome can occur, and is likely due to dopamine depletion. You may see symptoms such as choroid movements (wiggling or writhing), twitchiness, muscular contractions, restlessness, wiggling of hands and feet, or constant motion. They look a bit different from nervous movements since they have more of a fluid character.

Users can experience cardiac issues due to the constant excess of cate-cholamine release during stimulant use. Tachycardia may eventually cause cardiac muscle hypertrophy, leading to cardiomyopathy. Hypertension can occur, and there is an increased risk for myocardial infarction and stroke.

Lastly, "crack lung" is a sort of pulmonary allergic reaction to cocaine. It leads to shortness of breath, pleuritic chest pain, and infiltrates on a chest x-ray.

Withdrawal syndrome

Stimulants do not cause any obvious physical withdrawal syndromes, but they do cause fatigue, depression, irritability, and increased appetite, as well as suicidal behavior at times. There is no specific treatment for cocaine or other stimulant withdrawal. After several days, the symptoms go away on their own. These will be followed by cravings, which can be intense.

ASSESSMENT

As with all substance use assessments, ask your patients about the quantity and frequency of their stimulant use. Most people use stimulants in a binge pattern, and cravings are more prominent with stimulants than for many other drugs. Ask about associated symptoms, such as psychotic symptoms, paranoia, or depression.

For help with subsequent behavioral treatment, ask about how the drug is used. Often, environmental cues will trigger cravings. Since stimulants enhance alertness, everything that occurs around users while they are getting high is associated with that high. Triggers can be olfactory, such as the smell of fellow users' perfume or cologne, or tactile, such as the feeling of money in a pant or coat pocket.

To help motivate patients to make a behavior change, I ask about the consequences of their stimulant use. I may use the "good things/less-good things" technique or ask about a typical day (see Chapter 4). Consequences due to stimulant use may include interpersonal, financial, or legal effects. Stimulants are hard on the body and the mind, so there can be physical and mental health consequences. Because of the binge pattern of use, patients may spend a lot of money at a time on drugs, leading to significant financial difficulties.

CASE REVISITED: *N's pattern of cocaine use is mostly weekends. At an average of 2 days a week, she does not think she is addicted, but she acknowledges that she often chooses to spend time with cocaine-using friends rather than with her family. When pressed, she reports that sometimes her use is actually closer to 4 days a week, especially toward the beginning of the month when her boyfriend's paycheck arrives. When she uses, she spends $60/day. In addition to cocaine, N drinks 3–4 beers when she uses. She smokes marijuana sporadically, about 2–3 times per month, and also smokes a pack of cigarettes per day.*

Between episodes of cocaine use, N says she crashes and feels sad and disinterested. Once in a while, she has some psychotic symptoms, such as auditory hallucinations, during heavier binges. I diagnose her with cocaine use disorder, severe, based on symptoms of craving, more time spent on the drug than intended, problems with relationship, tolerance, and withdrawals.

TREATMENT

There is no pharmacotherapy for stimulant addiction, but frequently patients will have chronic depressive symptoms interrupted only by drug use. In these cases, antidepressants can be very helpful.

There's a saying in substance use treatment circles: "When you are trying to treat stimulants, the thing that works best is money." This refers to contingency management, which is essentially paying patients to quit (Lussier et al, 2006; McKay et al, 2010). While contingency management has been shown to be effective for most substance use disorders, I have found it particularly useful for stimulant use disorder.

Contingency management programs work in various ways, but their key element is identifying a group of behaviors that are likely to lead to lasting recovery, then rewarding people for these behaviors. Patients can be rewarded for negative urine drug tests, showing up to group or individual sessions, and completing therapy homework assignments. They can also be rewarded for consistency. For example, after several successive negative urine drug screens, their reward could increase.

The rewards themselves are usually not actual cash, but rather things like gift cards or lottery tickets. Research has shown that the chance of getting a big reward tends to be just as motivating as actually getting the reward—hence the common use of lottery tickets in programs. Contingency management is a way to enhance the outcomes of substance use treatment, but it can be expensive to implement. However, lottery tickets or small-denomination gift cards are less expensive and still work as motivational incentives, so contingency management can add value when used with other elements of a treatment program. Most early contingency management programs were funded as research programs, but now they are often subsidized by government grants or private donations.

Even though the rewards are not very large, they are more tangible than an abstract goal such as abstinence, and they give people an external motivation and keep them engaged in treatment. People will apply cognitive behavioral therapy skills in day-to-day life so they can accumulate skills to stay clean and get prizes. Eventually, the prizes become less important than the achievement of abstinence, and patients see the other benefits—their life rewards—take center stage.

CASE CONCLUSION: *After our evaluation session, N is in the contemplation stage of change. She recognizes there are problems with her cocaine use, but she maintains that she enjoys using. Her rationale is that her cocaine habit is how she connects to other people besides her family that are important to her.*

My tactic is to focus on her relationship with her boyfriend. There is a serious risk that he might leave her; in addition, she could lose custody of her son. N also recognizes the negative health effects of her drug use, since she has been told by her primary care physician that she is well on her way to developing high blood pressure and heart disease.

I also work to help N see the connection between her cocaine use and her depression. This makes sense to her, because she knows that her crashes cause her anhedonia. She also realizes that her poor mood lasts more than just a couple of days after a binge. Through her habit, she is chasing her tail—she uses coke, it makes her depressed, and then she uses coke because of depression. I help her realize that breaking that cycle will benefit her interpersonally, psychologically, and physically.

I decide to offer N contingency management. I start by telling her that at my clinic, patients can participate in prize drawings if they maintain clean urine screens and attend their sessions. When she expresses interest, I tell her that when patients give a negative urine sample, they can pull a chip out of a bag. About half of the chips have a monetary value, ranging from $5 to $100, and can be exchanged for a gift card to a store or a restaurant. As time goes on and patients succeed with urine testing, showing up to sessions and other activities, they get more picks from the bag. But if they miss a session or fail a urine test, they go back to just one pick.

N has weekly sessions with her therapist, and she graduates from contingency management after 3 months. She continues to apply the relapse prevention skills she has learned in cognitive behavioral therapy with the help of the contingency management rewards as motivation. After a while of practicing these, she eliminates her cocaine use. N is able to stay abstinent for a while and recognizes that the rewards of staying clean are even more valuable than the gift cards she's earned.

Self-Test Questions

1. A 32-year-old woman has been smoking crack cocaine once or twice a week for over 10 years. She is interested in quitting, but her previous quit attempts (on her own) have been unsuccessful. Which of the following treatments can you recommend to her as likely to be effective?
   a. Acamprosate
   b. Bupropion
   c. Contingency management
   d. Drug Abuse Resistance Education program

2. A 26-year-old man goes to a party at a friend's house and takes some amphetamine pills that are offered to him there. After using this drug, he is most likely to experience which of the following sets of symptoms?

    a. Nausea, muscle twitches, lacrimation, diarrhea

    b. Pupil dilation, tachycardia, hypertension, increased energy

    c. Slurred speech, ataxia, hypotension, vomiting

    d. Somnolence, pinpoint pupils, respiratory depression

3. A 23-year-old man is picked up by the police for erratic behavior in a public park and brought to the emergency department for evaluation. He is anxious; he believes that a late-night talk show host is putting thoughts into his mind, and he wants to leave before the "government gestapo" come to take him away. The man's vital signs are all elevated. He admits to using a substance at a party earlier that night. Which substance did he most likely use?

    a. Carbon tetrachloride

    b. Eszopiclone

    c. Gamma-hydroxybutyrate

    d. Methamphetamine

The answer key for these self-test questions is on page 233.

Note: If you purchased CME credit with this book, your CME post-test can be accessed when you are logged in at www.thecarlatreport.com/AddictionGuide. Please keep in mind that the question and answer order for that CME post-test are different than what you see in these self-test study questions.

CHAPTER 13

Designer Drugs

"I hate to advocate drugs, alcohol, violence, or insanity
to anyone, but they've always worked for me."

Hunter S. Thompson

TAKE HOME POINTS

- Newer designer drugs are not detected on current drug tests, and some contain compounds that are not illegal yet.
- Synthetic cannabinoids (spice) have effects similar to cannabis, but also have many more serious side effects.
- Synthetic cathinones (bath salts) are designer stimulants with potential for serious psychiatric and cardiovascular effects.
- Synthetic hallucinogens are associated with more cardiovascular effects and agitation than older classic hallucinogens.
- Treatment of acute intoxication with designer drugs is supportive.
- Long-term treatment of addiction to designer drugs is behavioral.

CASE VIGNETTE: *C is a 19-year-old male who started drinking alcohol and smoking cannabis on weekends in early high school with friends at parties. He had tried synthetic cannabinoids (spice), but found they made him more anxious than smoking cannabis (marijuana). About a year before I saw him, he was introduced to bath salts, which he snorted and vaped with his friends. C liked these more, because they made him awake and euphoric for late-night parties. A few months ago, one of his friends became agitated at a party, yelling at people to get away from him and saying zombies were trying to eat his brain. The police were called, and the friend was brought to an emergency room for treatment of transient psychosis due to cathinone ingestion. Despite promising his parents he* *would stop, C has continued to use bath salts and other drugs. His mother recently found a foil bath salts pouch in the house and insisted he seek treatment. C doesn't see using on weekends with his friends as problematic.*

Designer drugs represent a new and dangerous trend in drug development. They are analogues of other drugs, designed and produced in clandestine laboratories, developed specifically to avoid detection and prosecution by law authorities. Because they are slightly different in chemical structure, they are (currently) legal because the DEA has not yet officially categorized them as banned Schedule I substances. They are typically marketed as "legal highs" with effects comparable to cannabis, stimulants, or hallucinogens. Designer drugs are often sold on the internet, where they are advertised as "plant food" or "research chemicals" that are "not for human consumption." Most cannot be detected on standard drug screens.

The term "club drugs" was coined by the National Institute on Drug Abuse to identify drugs commonly used on the club scene, such as dance parties, raves, and circuit parties. Although there is some overlap between designer drugs and club drugs, most of the popular club drugs, such as ecstasy (MDMA) and LSD, are well-known illicit substances and are classified as Schedule I drugs by the DEA. See Chapter 14 for more information on club drugs.

There are three main categories of designer drugs: synthetic cannabinoids, synthetic cathinones (stimulants), and synthetic hallucinogens.

SYNTHETIC CANNABINOIDS

Sold as "spice," "K2," or "incense," synthetic cannabinoids allow people to achieve a cannabis-like high for a lower price and without risking detection by commonly administered urine drug screens. While many people assume these products are herbs that naturally produce intoxication, in fact they are usually inert herbs sprayed with various THC analogues.

Synthetic cannabinoids originated from basic research on cannabinoid agonists. For example, a popular group of cannabinoids is called "JWH-018," "JWH-073," and various other names. The JWH comes from the name of a prominent professor of organic chemistry at Clemson University, John W. Huffman. Beginning in 1984, Huffman and colleagues developed over 450 cannabinoid analogues in hopes of developing treatments for multiple sclerosis, HIV/AIDS, and cancer. In the 2000s, some of these compounds began to show up in Europe as recreational drugs, and they quickly spread to the U.S.

> **FUN FACT: Why Is It Called "Spice"?**
> The street name "spice" for early varieties of synthetic cannabinoids refers to the mind-altering, life-prolonging spice mélange that made space travel possible in the science fiction novel *Dune* by Frank Herbert. Now all synthetic cannabinoids are referred to as spice, regardless of branding.

The chemicals found in these drugs are generally cannabinoid agonists that have significantly more potency at the CB1 and CB2 receptors than THC. For example, HU-210 (so named because it was developed at Hebrew University) is up to 800 times more potent. The various products sold as herbal incense are cocktails of diverse chemicals, both THC analogues and other designer compounds, and it's impossible to know what one is ingesting with any given product—which is one of the dangers.

The psychotropic effects of synthetic cannabinoids are very similar to cannabis, such as euphoria, heightened perceptions, time distortion, and others. But because of their much higher potency, they also confer a higher risk of negative side effects, including anxiety, paranoia, hypertension, and tachycardia (Weaver et al, 2015). In addition, because some of the products may contain even more dangerous compounds, such as cathinones (more on these later), there have been cases of life-threatening or fatal effects, including seizure, renal failure, toxic hepatitis, cardiac ischemia, and stroke.

Withdrawal syndromes

As is sometimes the case with heavy cannabis users (see Chapter 10), regular users of synthetic cannabinoids develop tolerance as well as withdrawal symptoms. The withdrawal symptoms and time course are similar to cannabis (5–7 days of irritability, insomnia, anxiety, depression, nausea, vomiting, and headache). The only treatment is supportive, though since there is cross-tolerance between cannabis and synthetic cannabinoids, either can substitute for the other as a means for patients to end withdrawal symptoms. Naturally, this defeats the purpose of trying to treat the withdrawal syndrome because it just delays the inevitable onset of withdrawal symptoms.

Assessment

When talking to patients, ask directly about synthetic cannabinoid products and use several names (see Table 13-1 later in the chapter), since not all users will be aware of their various names and slang terms. Use is more likely in patients who already use cannabis or other types of designer drugs, those who are younger (teenagers and young adults), and those who may have specific reasons to avoid detection on urine drug tests (those on probation, in the military, or who have workplace drug testing).

Since synthetic cannabinoids and other recent designer drugs are not detected by routine drug screens, health care providers who rely only on laboratory testing may be fooled into believing illicit drugs have not been used. Conversely, the presence of routinely detectable illicit substances does not rule out the presence of designer drugs, since polysubstance use is typical in designer drug users.

If a patient admits to synthetic cannabinoid use, then ask follow-up questions about amount used, frequency of use, and recent pattern of use. Also ask about drug effects, both pleasurable and adverse.

Treatment

There are no specific treatments for synthetic cannabinoid use, as there is no specific treatment for cannabis use disorder. In emergency rooms, patients who've smoked too much spice or similar substances can present with anxiety, agitation, or paranoia. The best approach is to keep the user in a quiet environment until the acute effects subside, usually within 2–6 hours. Long-term treatment involves standard substance use treatment techniques such as motivational interviewing, cognitive behavioral therapy, and 12-step programs.

SYNTHETIC CATHINONES

Known on the street as "bath salts," synthetic cathinones are more potent derivatives of the active ingredient in khat (*Catha edulis*), a plant traditionally chewed for its stimulant properties in parts of Africa and the Arabian Peninsula. Most bath salt products contain a mixture of synthetic cathinones, including methylenedioxypyrovalerone (MDPV), methylone, and mephedrone. Methylone and mephedrone are amphetamine-like chemicals in the monoamine system, while MDPV is a cocaine-like blocker of

> ⭕ **CLINICAL PEARL: Asking About Designer Drug Use**
> - *Have you ever tried . . . [list names of local designer drugs]?*
> - *Which drugs do you like to use together?*
> - *How do you like to use that drug? Do you smoke, snort, or inject intravenously?*
> - *Have you ever had a bad trip or a bad reaction to one of those drugs?*
> - *Have any of your friends had a bad trip from those drugs?*
> - *Have you or one of your friends had to go to the emergency department for a bad trip?*
> - *Are you using more now than before? Why?*
> - *Do you have cravings?*
> - *Have you tried to cut down or quit?*

monoamine reuptake. Interestingly, the antidepressant bupropion is also a cathinone derivative.

Bath salts usually appear as a crystalline powder that can be swallowed, snorted, or injected. Since they are chemically related to methamphetamine and ecstasy, it's no surprise they can cause dangerously high blood pressure, stroke, myocardial infarction, hyperthermia, psychosis, aggression, and other severe complications in those who ingest them (Capriola, 2013).

Withdrawal syndromes

As with other stimulants, bath salts do not have an obvious physical withdrawal syndrome. Users will develop tolerance to bath salt effects with regular use, and withdrawal symptoms are basically the opposite of effects of intoxication, including irritability, depression, somnolence, and increased appetite. Additional effects reported with bath salt withdrawal include difficulty concentrating, nasal congestion, and insomnia. These symptoms usually last for 2–3 days. There is no specific treatment for withdrawal from bath salts, just supportive care with rest and adequate hydration.

Assessment and treatment

Since bath salts are not detected by standard drug screens, the primary way of assessing use is by asking patients. Emergency room doctors will see some patients with acute agitation, and—more ominously—tachycardia, elevated blood pressure, and chest pain. Common emergency treatments are symptomatic and include benzodiazepines and antipsychotics.

CASE REVISITED: *I talk with C about what benefits he is getting from using bath salts. He only uses them with his friends at weekend parties. In terms of less-good things, he recognizes that his parents are concerned about his health and that continuing to party all night may jeopardize being able to live in his parents' house. After his friend's "zombie incident," C has started thinking more seriously about the possible risks of using bath salts. I ask him what else he thinks could happen, then give him some general feedback about complications of bath salt use. He agrees to think about the subject some more and talk with his parents.*

SYNTHETIC HALLUCINOGENS

Soon after the DEA banned several "bath salt" compounds in 2011, clandestine chemists began manufacturing and marketing a new chemical: 4-iodo-2,5dimethoxy-N-(2-methoxybenzyl) phenethylamine. This compound—more efficiently referred to as 25I-NBOMe, N-bomb, "smiles," and other clever monikers—is a high-affinity 5HT2A agonist that causes hallucinatory experiences like those produced by LSD or psilocybin. As with LSD, the most common way of ingesting N-bomb is via blotter paper placed under the tongue. See Chapter 14 for more on the effects of LSD.

The typical desired effects are nearly identical to LSD—psychedelic visions, enhanced colors, a sense of euphoric connectedness, and so on. Unfortunately, N-bombs are nowhere near as "safe" as their older serotonergic relatives. Many users experience psychiatric consequences that require medical attention. These include dysphoria, confusion, agitation, aggression, paranoia, and self-harm behaviors that go far beyond what has been observed among users of more traditional hallucinogens over many decades (Weaver et al, 2015).

As if psychiatric consequences weren't enough, a potentially lethal serotonergic toxidrome known as "excited delirium" has also been described. This includes agitation, tachycardia, hypertension, and hyperthermia, and it has been associated with several deaths. There have been several case reports of dramatic suicides in association with 25I-NBOMe (Suzuki et al, 2014).

TABLE 13-1. Common Designer Drugs: Useful Information

Category	Names[1]	Active Ingredients[2]	Pharmacology	How Taken	Effects/Toxicity	Tolerance/ Withdrawal	Clinical Testing Available?
Synthetic cannabinoids	**Spice, K2, incense,** Kannabliss, King Cobra, Black Diamond, Stona Lisa, and many more (see http:// www.spice4fun.com)	JWH-018, JWH-073, JWH-200, CP-47,497, (C8)-CP-47,497, and others	CB1 receptor agonist	Smoking or vaping	Euphoria, anxiety, agitation, psychosis, tachycardia, seizures, myocardial infarction	Yes	Yes, but not widely available
Synthetic cathinones	**Bath salts, flakka,** plant food, jewelry cleaner, chicken food additive, research chemical, MCAT, meow, ivory wave, Ivory Coast, and many more	MDPV, methylone, mephedrone, and others	Inhibit reuptake of serotonin, norepinephrine, and dopamine	Oral ingestion, snorting, and vaping	Euphoria, agitation, severe hypertension, psychosis, rage episodes, agitated delirium syndrome, myocarditis, rhabdomyolysis, renal failure, death	Yes	Yes, but not widely available
Synthetic hallucinogens	**N-Bomb,** en-bomb, smile, 25I, 25B, 25C	25I-NBOMe	Serotonin agonist	Absorbed through mucous membranes (think "blotter acid")	Hallucinations, paranoia, suicidal panic, stabbing self and others, hypertension, tachycardia, seizures	Tolerance, but not withdrawal	Yes, but not widely available

[1]Most common street names in boldface

[2]Active ingredients listed so that you can recognize (or request) lab results for particular compounds

Withdrawal syndromes

Like all hallucinogens, synthetic designer drugs such as NBOMe do not have a discrete withdrawal syndrome. Tolerance to the recreational effects develops rapidly with repeated use, but abrupt discontinuation does not produce significant ill effects.

Assessment and treatment

On physical exam, enlarged pupils are a sign of hallucinogen intoxication. Physiologic effects are more likely with NBOMe and other synthetic hallucinogens than most classic hallucinogens. Elevated heart rate and blood pressure are commonly seen, although nonspecific, but can provide a clue to distinguish use of more modern hallucinogens from older ones. Very brisk reflexes can be elicited. Seizures are also more likely than with older hallucinogens.

As with the other designer drugs, there is no treatment for either acute intoxication or long-term use, other than supportive care and traditional substance abuse counseling and programming.

CASE CONCLUSION: *After thinking about things and talking with his parents, C is more willing to enter treatment for his addictions. I discuss with him that bath salts themselves are risky, and combining them with alcohol, tobacco, and cannabis is also likely to lead to future problems. I refer him to a therapist for individual counseling, who also conducts some family counseling with C and his parents. I encourage C's parents to go to some Nar-Anon meetings, where they meet other parents of polysubstance-using teenagers. C is able to stop using illicit drugs and reduces his use of alcohol dramatically. He is now thinking of going to community college, and his parents are supportive of this.*

Self-Test Questions

1. A 16-year-old male is brought to the emergency department by his parents when he displays symptoms of anxiety and paranoia. Earlier in the evening, he had smoked a new drug; he shows the attending physician a packet with a colorful label that says the packet contains "bath salts." This type of substance belongs in which of the following drug classes?

a. Sedatives
b. Opioids
c. Stimulants
d. Cannabinoids

2. You are asked to evaluate a 15-year-old boy who is agitated and very frightened by what he says is a monster in his closet that wants to eat him. The boy admits to you that earlier in the day he tried a substance with his older friends. Except for a rapid heart rate, his vital signs are normal. His physical exam is also normal, except for bilateral prominent conjunctival blood vessels. This boy most likely used which of the following substances?
a. Amyl nitrite
b. Dextromethorphan
c. Mephedrone
d. Synthetic cannabinoid

3. Which of the following designer drugs has been associated with a serotonergic "excited delirium"?
a. 25I-NBOMe
b. Cathinone
c. JWH-018
d. Methylone

The answer key for these self-test questions is on page 233.

Note: If you purchased CME credit with this book, your CME post-test can be accessed when you are logged in at www.thecarlatreport.com/AddictionGuide. Please keep in mind that the question and answer order for that CME post-test are different than what you see in these self-test study questions.

CHAPTER 14

Hallucinogens and Other Drugs

"If God dropped acid, would he see people?"
Steven Wright, comedian

TAKE HOME POINTS

- Hallucinogens include LSD, psilocybin, mescaline, and others.
- Club drugs include MDMA, ketamine, methamphetamine, and others.
- Dissociative drugs include PCP and ketamine.
- Most of these drugs are used sporadically and cause neither physical dependence nor withdrawal syndromes.
- They are commonly used in conjunction with cannabis, alcohol, and other substances.

CASE VIGNETTE: *B is a 27-year-old unemployed male who presents with the desire to get his drug use under control. Around age 14 he became a regular smoker of marijuana, and at age 16 he started using LSD and psilocybin and would also use MDMA (ecstasy) periodically. In his early 20s, he was introduced to IV ketamine, which he used heavily for several months until he had a psychotic episode and was admitted to a psychiatric hospital. He was treated with Haldol and returned to his baseline mental status within a week; it was clear to both B and the attending physician that his psychosis was induced by ketamine use. Thereafter, he continued intermittent use of cannabis and hallucinogens. B has been unable to keep a job, is often homeless, and has been in and out of jail for trespassing, breaking and entering, and petty theft (which finances his drug use). When he sees me, he says he is "burning out" and wants to "get his life together."*

Introduction

I've grouped hallucinogens with club drugs and inhalants, because all three types of drugs tend to be used sporadically, often in social situations (see Table 14-1). They don't produce prominent physical dependence or withdrawal syndromes. Often, people use them opportunistically—meaning, for example, with other users at a party or rave. When used infrequently, they rarely cause problems, and you will be unlikely to see people who are exclusively addicted to specific hallucinogens. However, some people use these drugs frequently, often mixing and matching them with a variety of similar drugs.

CLASSIC HALLUCINOGENS: LSD AND OTHERS

The classic hallucinogens include LSD, psilocybin, mescaline, and a few others that are less well-known. They all cause similar effects and are all relatively safe—at least compared to the dissociative drugs like PCP and ketamine, or the newer designer drugs (see Chapter 13).

The subjective effects of hallucinogens vary widely. Most commonly, users will notice perceptual distortions, ranging from enhanced sensations to visual changes to outright hallucination. Common visual effects include changes in colors, light trails behind moving objects, and multiple images of a single object. Synesthesias, or cross-linking of senses, may occur; for example, people may "smell" colors and "taste" sounds. Some people report various dissociative sensations, such as feeling that their bodies are separated from their environments.

Existential insights are an important part of the hallucinogenic experience. Users often have an epic sense of feeling at one with the universe, being connected to all of humanity, and feeling they are about to meet God.

Potential negative effects of hallucinogens include intense anxiety, a sense of doom, or knowledge of the impending death of oneself or the world, with ominous hallucinations such as melting walls and crumbling cities. A "bad trip" refers to a prolonged, overwhelming anxiety attack, which can occur unpredictably. Any hallucinogen can cause a bad trip, although some are more likely than others to do so, especially phencyclidine.

Here's a more specific rundown of the hallucinogens you may hear about from patients.

Lysergic acid diethylamide (LSD)

LSD was the original "acid" and was first synthesized in 1938 by Albert

TABLE 14-1. Hallucinogens

Drug	Source	Street Name(s)	Brand Name
Alpha-methyltryptamine (AMT)	Synthetic	Love pills, trip	Indopan
Bromo-dimethoxyphenethylamine (2-CB)	Synthetic	Bromo, DOB, nexus, spectrum	Erox
Bufotenine	Colorado river toad venom	Bufo, toad-licking	
Diisopropyl-methoxytryptamine (MeO-DIPT)	Synthetic	Foxy, foxy-methoxy	
Dimethoxymethyl-amphetamine (DOM)	Synthetic	STP (Serenity, Tranquility, and Peace)	
Dimethoxy-propylthiophenethylamine (2C-T-7)	Synthetic	7-Up, tripstacy, blue mystic	
Dimethyltryptamine (DMT)	Canary grass, prairie bundleflower, caapi vine	Dimitri, businessman's trip, ayahuasca, fantasia	
Flunitrazepam	Synthetic	Roofies	Rohypnol
Gamma-hydroxybutyrate (GHB)	Synthetic	Georgia Home Boy, Grievous Bodily Harm	Xyrem
Ibogaine	West African iboga shrub	Ibo, iboga	
Ibotinic acid, muscinol	Mushrooms		
Ketamine	Synthetic	Special K, kit cat, cat valium	Ketalar
Lysergic acid diethylamide (LSD)	Synthetic	Acid, blotter, microdot	
Lysergic acid hydroxyethylamide (LSA)	Morning glory seeds, Hawaiian baby woodrose	Natural high, organic high	
Mescaline	Peyote cactus	Mesc, peyote, cactus	
Methamphetamine	Synthetic	Meth, crank, speed, uppers	Desoxyn
Methylenedioxy-amphetamine (MDA)	Synthetic	The love drug, Eve	
Methylenedioxy-methamphetamine (MDMA)	Synthetic	Ecstasy, X, Adam	
Phencyclidine (PCP)	Synthetic	Angel dust, PeaCe Pill	Sernyl
Psilocybin	Mushrooms	Magic mushrooms, shrooms	
Salvinorin-A	Salvia divinorum (Diviner's sage)	Salvia, Sallie D	

Hoffman, a chemist at Sandoz Laboratories (now Novartis) in Switzerland. Hoffman was the first person to ingest LSD—initially by accident—and in 1943 he described his experience thusly: *"At home I lay down and sank into a not unpleasant intoxicated-like condition, characterized by an extremely stimulated imagination. In a dreamlike state, with eyes closed (I found the daylight to be unpleasantly glaring), I perceived an uninterrupted stream of fantastic pictures, extraordinary shapes with intense, kaleidoscopic play of colors. After some two hours this condition faded away."*

LSD became a popular recreational drug in the 1960s, when it became a symbol of the counterculture. It is now widely available, and is usually sold as drops of liquid saturated into blotter paper, which is then placed on the tongue and absorbed into the mucous membranes. The effects begin within 20 minutes and last a few hours.

> **FUN FACT: LSD and Rye Bread**
> The original source for LSD was rye fungus. LSD was initially synthesized from lysergic acid found in ergot, a fungus that grows on rye and other types of grain.

Psilocybin

Psilocybin is a hallucinogenic compound produced by many species of mushrooms. The prolific Albert Hoffman led a research team that identified psilocybin as the psychoactive compound in those mushrooms. It is sold as dried mushrooms, which are eaten. The onset of effects is within 30 minutes and lasts 3–4 hours, and its subjective effects are very similar to LSD.

Mescaline

Mescaline occurs naturally in the peyote cactus, as well as some other cactus species. It has been used in Native American tribal ceremonies for centuries. On the street, it is often sold as a liquid which is ingested. Its effects and time course are similar to other hallucinogens, though it is more amphetamine-like and causes elevations in pulse and blood pressure.

Other hallucinogens

Many hallucinogens with effects similar to LSD have been synthesized and marketed, such as the following:

• DMT (dimethyltryptamine), otherwise known as Dimitri or businessman's trip. This is essentially a very short-acting version of LSD. It lasts about an hour, hence its nickname "businessman's trip," referring to the fact that one could theoretically drop DMT during lunch and be clearheaded in time for the first afternoon meeting.

- Mescaline derivatives: STP, MDA, DMA, MDMA. All of these agents provide hallucinogenic highs combined with amphetamine effects. By far the most popular of these is MDMA, or ecstasy, which we'll cover in detail later in the chapter.

Treatment

CASE CONCLUSION: *I diagnose B with depression and prescribe him an SSRI. In addition, I refer him to a therapeutic community run by the Salvation Army. The therapeutic community proves a good fit for B. His mood improves, and he is able to maintain sobriety.*

People occasionally show up in emergency rooms with acute panic as a result of a bad trip, and in these cases providing a rapid-acting benzodiazepine like alprazolam or lorazepam is the cornerstone of treatment. For patients with temporary hallucinogen-induced psychosis, an antipsychotic may be needed in addition to a benzodiazepine.

For long-term treatment of hallucinogen use disorder, you will usually be treating comorbid psychiatric problems, such as major depression or schizophrenia. In B's case, his long history of polysubstance use has led to stagnation and homelessness, and therefore he needs a therapeutic community in addition to individual treatment. Therapeutic communities (see Chapter 3) are extended residential programs usually run by a faith-based nonprofit and supported by donations. They are often populated by homeless men with drug issues. The residents may be given various kinds of work training, such as working in a Salvation Army thrift shop. Staff at the program can teach residents skills of living, like making a resume and preparing for a job. These programs usually include Narcotics Anonymous meetings. The placements can be long-term, and clients may stay for many years and eventually work as peer counselors.

CLUB DRUGS

CASE VIGNETTE: *R, an 18-year-old male high school graduate but since unemployed, is referred by his parents, who've told him he must get* *treatment if he wants to keep living at home. As a younger teen, R smoked marijuana, binge drank, and used mushrooms and LSD fairly regularly with his friends. Several months ago, he was introduced to MDMA and began taking it 2–3 times per week, usually at raves. He had several subsequent experiences of crashing, in which he felt severely depressed and would spend a day or two in his room. R experimented with other drugs as well. At one party, he snorted some bath salts and had a panic attack. Another time, he found a packet of powder in his wallet that he decided to snort, even though he didn't recognize what it was. As a result, he blacked out over an entire weekend, and people later told him that he had done and said strange things. His parents are fed up; they have stopped paying R's phone bill and no longer allow him to use the family car. Because he feels trapped in the house with his parents, R agrees to be evaluated.*

A "club drug" is a classification first coined by the National Institute on Drug Abuse to identify drugs commonly used on the club scene, especially at raves. (Raves, or circuit parties, are all-night dance parties held in warehouses or basements of nightclubs.)

MDMA

MDMA (ecstasy) was first synthesized in 1912 by chemists at Merck who were trying to develop a drug to stop abnormal bleeding. Not much happened with the drug until the 1970s, when a prominent chemist named Alexander Shulgin discovered it and began to publish about it in the scientific literature. Psychotherapists soon learned about MDMA and used it as an adjunct to psychotherapy. Gradually, it filtered out into the club scene and

FUN FACT: Dr. Ecstasy

Alexander Shulgin was a biochemist who worked for Dow Chemicals during most of his career. He developed an early interest in the chemistry of hallucinogens and synthesized over 200 psychoactive compounds. He tested each compound on himself, and is famous for a self-published textbook describing the subjective effects of each molecule, *PiHKAL: A Chemical Love Story* (PiHKAL is short for "Phenethylamines I Have Known and Loved"). (http://www.nytimes.com/2005/01/30/magazine/dr-ecstasy.html)

became one of the defining drugs of raves. Recently, there has been a renewal of MDMA research for psychiatric treatment, with promising results in the treatment of PTSD (Tupper et al, 2015).

MDMA produces a sense of euphoria and a desire to connect with others, including a desire to touch others, though not in a sexual way. Its amphetamine-like properties produce an increase in energy and a decreased need for sleep. After MDMA's effects wear off, there is often a significant crash with fatigue and a sense of depression.

Physical effects include an increase in muscle tension, heart rate, blood pressure, and body temperature. Dangerous dehydration can occur if high doses are taken, especially in the setting of a rave where people are dancing vigorously in a room with many other warm bodies. Potential electrolyte abnormalities and rhabdomyolysis (muscle breakdown) can occur at any time and may lead to acute kidney failure. MDMA appears to temporarily deplete the brain of serotonin, which can lead to feelings of depression after use, though it's unclear whether this actually damages the brain. Several studies suggest MDMA use can lead to cognitive decline in otherwise healthy young people, even at typical recreational doses (Gouzoulis-Mayfrank et al, 2000).

Dissociative anesthetics

PCP (phencyclidine)

Also known as "angel dust," PCP is a veterinary anesthetic (hence the term "horse tranquilizer"). It was originally used in humans as well, but it caused such profound out-of-body experiences that patients sometimes felt they were floating above their bodies and looking down at themselves when emerging from deep anesthesia after surgery (known as an "emergence reaction"). This led to significant anxiety, and therefore its use in humans was discontinued.

PCP is usually snorted or injected. Some users dip a cannabis joint into a PCP solution, called "embalming fluid" or "fry," and then smoke it. The drug's effects begin in 20–30 minutes and last longer than most hallucinogens, generally 6–8 hours. PCP leads to a range of subjective effects. Because it is like taking a sedative, an amphetamine, and a hallucinogen all at once, people feel drunk, accelerated, and dissociated. And since PCP is an anesthetic, users also tend to be pain-insensitive. The caricature of the highly aggressive and agitated PCP user—think of the movie *The Terminator*—has some accuracy, particularly at very high doses.

FUN FACT: MDMA and Raves

Raves are at the center of an underground culture that is organized around MDMA and other club drugs. Organizers will publicize the raves by putting up flyers with "E" (for ecstasy) prominently displayed. Participants can purchase MDMA at the party, though it is sometimes substituted with other drugs. Ecstasy test kits are available to test the purity of drugs on the spot. The music at a rave is typically techno, which is wordless music with a driving beat. People bring glow sticks because various hallucinogen-like club drugs, especially MDMA, allow you to see light trails. There are designer pacifiers, often neon-colored, for people to wear to minimize bruxism (jaw clenching), a common side effect of MDMA.

Ketamine

Also known as "Special K," ketamine is FDA-approved as an anesthetic agent and is primarily used for children and in veterinary medicine. It has also been the focus of recent psychiatric attention because several randomized controlled trials have shown that intravenous ketamine is an effective rapid treatment of depression.

Recreational users snort or inject ketamine and experience trance-like states and hallucinatory out-of-body experiences. Many of these experiences are so distinct that they have specific names. "Transformations" refer to a sensation that one's body is made of a different substance, like wood or rubber. "Complete separation" refers to feeling totally separated from one's body. This is also called being in a "K-hole," because users feel like they are at the bottom of a well looking up at their body.

Ketamine does not last as long as PCP, and its effects are somewhat gentler.

Club sedatives

GHB (gamma hydroxybutyrate) is a sedative marketed for the treatment of narcolepsy under the brand name Xyrem. It has gained popularity on the club scene because it causes mild euphoria and relaxation, much like a stiff drink or benzodiazepines. At high doses it is dangerous and can lead to vomiting, loss of consciousness, and seizure. It can also cause amnesia, leading to blackouts; as such it is sometimes used as a date rape drug, since the victim may not remember the sexual assault.

Flunitrazepam (Rohypnol) is a benzodiazepine which is also sometimes used as a date rape drug, although this seems to be rare. It is an odorless, colorless solution that can be surreptitiously added to a potential victim's drink, and its effects are synergistic with alcohol.

Inhalants

Inhalants are a very diverse group of chemical compounds, which are inhaled or "huffed" in order to obtain a very brief high that is a little like an alcohol buzz. Many common household items can be used as inhalants. They include air dusters, epoxies such as model airplane glue, and a variety of hydrocarbons such as butane lighter fluid, gasoline, paint thinner, and other cleaning solvents.

Nitrous oxide, used in dental procedures and often referred to as "laughing gas," is a popular inhalant. Although it can be obtained on the black market for recreational use, small amounts of nitrous oxide are used as propellants for many types of spray cans (ie, whipped cream, hair spray), and users can inhale small amounts by pressing the nozzles. Freon from air conditioner units is also siphoned off and inhaled, and is nicknamed "Freebies."

FUN FACT: 19th-Century Inhalants

In the 1840s, "ether frolics" involved the inhalation of ether at parties, which were often held by medical students.

Inhalants are popular with younger people because they are easy to obtain and produce a short high. In addition, legal penalties are almost nonexistent compared with possession of illegal drugs.

Certain inhalants are popular in the gay community as enhancements to sexual activity—these include nitric oxide and butyl nitrite, with nicknames such as "aroma of men" and "locker room" (referencing their smell, which is like sweaty socks). Butyl and amyl nitrite are available in head shops (stores that sell paraphernalia such as water pipes, e-cigarettes, or vaporizers for use of tobacco or cannabis products) and come in plastic capsules that users pop open to sniff, hence their street name "poppers."

Because they are industrial solvents and other compounds not meant for human consumption, inhalants are dangerous. They can lead to hypoxia since they displace oxygen, and can cause arrhythmias, brain damage, and death. Those who huff chronically are vulnerable to liver damage, kidney failure, peripheral neuropathy, and early dementia.

In talking to kids about inhalants, I emphasize that they are playing with fire and engaging in a practice that's more dangerous than they might realize. I'll tell parents to look for discolorations or sores around the nose and mouth, which are caused by skin irritation or pigmentation from inhaling and are a clue to their children's habits.

Assessment

When asking about hallucinogens, I'll use the typical normalization method: "Many people have tried things like LSD or PCP (acid or angel dust). Have you tried that or anything like it?" If the patient says "no," I'll give other examples, like shrooms or ecstasy.

Another important question is frequency of use: Is it regular, or just experimental? It's pretty rare for people to be long-term exclusive hallucinogen users; hallucinogens are more commonly used in the context of smoking pot or drinking.

I'll also ask, "How often do you have a bad trip?" It lets me get my foot in the door in terms of finding a way to motivate patients to decrease their use.

Treatment

Opportunistic (sporadic) users will often mature out of the use of these drugs. In more frequent users, I look for untreated depression and maladaptive coping skills. Adolescent-focused intensive outpatient programs can be helpful, though they are not easy to find. These programs teach healthier ways of dealing with life's problems.

Many hallucinogen users are young and lack insight, especially if they don't have rewarding experiences outside of drug use. They can be challenging to work with. I try to be very concrete and directive with assignments.

CASE CONCLUSION: *Initially, R is not particularly motivated to address his drug use, since he feels like he's been forced into treatment by his parents. Nonetheless, I give him the assignment to read parts of the Narcotics Anonymous "Big Book" and to write a half page every day about his reactions to it. This ends up being a useful exercise. R reads about other people's* *experiences that are similar to his own. He recognizes that they, like him, have experienced the consequences as well as the pleasures of substance abuse. He learns about other people's moments of clarity and about how they've learned to enjoy life by being clean. R starts to feel remorse for what he has put his parents through, and he reduces his drug use. As he improves, his parents loosen their grip on his privileges, which is positive. R gets involved in a student recovery group at a community college, which also helps him in his recovery.*

Self-Test Questions

1. A 13-year-old girl is brought in by her mother for evaluation of occasional confusion and clumsiness, as well as a one-year history of headaches that have progressed to daily and resulted in missing days from school. Her grades have declined significantly over the past school semester. On physical examination, the patient's lips and perioral area are dry and cracked, there are some sores on her chin, and her fingernail beds appear stained with ink. Which of the following substances has this girl most likely been using?
   a. Isopropanol (rubbing alcohol)
   b. Ketamine
   c. Meperidine
   d. Toluene

2. A 17-year-old girl is referred by her parents due to a marked drop in grades over the recent school semester; her parents express concern that she sometimes seems "spaced out." When asked routine screening questions about substance use, she admits to using alpha-methyltryptamine with a friend over the past few months. The patient agrees that she does not want these consequences. Which of the following treatment modalities is most appropriate for this patient?
   a. Individual and group counseling
   b. Aversion therapy
   c. Maintenance pharmacotherapy
   d. Drug Abuse Resistance Education program

3. Which of the following has been labeled a "club drug" by the National Institute on Drug Abuse (NIDA)?

a. Phencyclidine (PCP)

b. Gamma hydroxybutyrate (GHB)

c. Dextromethorphan (Robitussin)

d. Methylphenidate (Ritalin)

The answer key for these self-test questions is on page 233.

Note: If you purchased CME credit with this book, your CME post-test can be accessed when you are logged in at www.thecarlatreport.com/AddictionGuide. Please keep in mind that the question and answer order for that CME post-test are different than what you see in these self-test study questions.

Appendix

CLINICAL INSTITUTE WITHDRAWAL ASSESSMENT OF ALCOHOL SCALE, REVISED (CIWA-AR)

AUTHOR'S NOTE: *The Clinical Institute Withdrawal Assessment of Alcohol Scale is primarily used for documenting the severity of alcohol withdrawal syndrome in inpatients undergoing detox. It is useful for outpatient providers in that it is a reminder of the type and severity of symptoms seen in alcohol withdrawal.*

Patient: _____

Date: _____ Time: _____ (24 hour clock, midnight = 00:00)

Pulse or heart rate, taken for one minute: _____

Blood pressure: _____

NAUSEA AND VOMITING — Ask "Do you feel sick to your stomach? Have you vomited?" Observation.
 0 no nausea and no vomiting
 1 mild nausea with no vomiting
 2
 3
 4 intermittent nausea with dry heaves
 5
 6
 7 constant nausea, frequent dry heaves and vomiting

TACTILE DISTURBANCES — Ask "Have you any itching, pins and needles sensations, any burning, any numbness, or do you feel bugs crawling on or under your skin?" Observation.
 0 none
 1 very mild itching, pins and needles, burning or numbness
 2 mild itching, pins and needles, burning or numbness
 3 moderate itching, pins and needles, burning or numbness
 4 moderately severe hallucinations
 5 severe hallucinations
 6 extremely severe hallucinations
 7 continuous hallucinations

TREMOR — Arms extended and fingers spread apart. Observation.

0   no tremor

1   not visible, but can be felt fingertip to fingertip

2

3

4   moderate, with patient's arms extended

5

6

7   severe, even with arms not extended

AUDITORY DISTURBANCES — Ask "Are you more aware of sounds around you? Are they harsh? Do they frighten you? Are you hearing anything that is disturbing to you? Are you hearing things you know are not there?" Observation.

0   not present

1   very mild harshness or ability to frighten

2   mild harshness or ability to frighten

3   moderate harshness or ability to frighten

4   moderately severe hallucinations

5   severe hallucinations

6   extremely severe hallucinations

7   continuous hallucinations

PAROXYSMAL SWEATS — Observation.

0   no sweat visible

1   barely perceptible sweating, palms moist

2

3

4   beads of sweat obvious on forehead

5

6

7   drenching sweats

VISUAL DISTURBANCES — Ask "Does the light appear to be too bright? Is its color different? Does it hurt your eyes? Are you seeing anything that is disturbing to you? Are you seeing things you know are not there?" Observation.

0   not present

1   very mild sensitivity

2   mild sensitivity

3   moderate sensitivity

4   moderately severe hallucinations

5 severe hallucinations

6 extremely severe hallucinations

7 continuous hallucinations

ANXIETY — Ask "Do you feel nervous?" Observation.

0 no anxiety, at ease

1 mild anxious

2

3

4 moderately anxious, or guarded, so anxiety is inferred

5

6

7 equivalent to acute panic states as seen in severe delirium or acute schizophrenic reactions

HEADACHE, FULLNESS IN HEAD — Ask "Does your head feel different? Does it feel like there is a band around your head?" Do not rate for dizziness or lightheadedness. Otherwise, rate severity.

0 not present

1 very mild

2 mild

3 moderate

4 moderately severe

5 severe

6 very severe

7 extremely severe

ORIENTATION AND CLOUDING OF SENSORIUM — Ask "What day is this? Where are you? Who am I?"

0 oriented and can do serial additions

1 cannot do serial additions or is uncertain about date

2 disoriented for date by no more than 2 calendar days

3 disoriented for date by more than 2 calendar days

4 disoriented for place/or person

AGITATION — Observation.

0 normal activity

1 somewhat more than normal activity

2

3

4 moderately fidgety and restless

5

6

7 paces back and forth during most of the interview, or constantly thrashes
about

Total **CIWA-Ar** Score _____

_____ Rater's Initials

Maximum Possible Score 67

The **CIWA-Ar** is not copyrighted and may be reproduced freely. This assessment for monitoring withdrawal symptoms requires approximately 5 minutes to administer. The maximum score is 67 (see instrument). Patients scoring less than 10 do not usually need additional medication for withdrawal.

Sullivan, J.T.; Sykora, K.; Schneiderman, J.; Naranjo, C.A.; and Sellers, E.M. Assessment of alcohol withdrawal: The revised Clinical Institute Withdrawal Assessment for Alcohol scale (**CIWA-Ar**). *British Journal of Addiction* 84:1353-1357, 1989.

CLINICAL OPIATE WITHDRAWAL SCALE

AUTHOR'S NOTE: *The Clinical Opiate Withdrawal Scale (COWS) is an 11-item scale designed to be administered by a clinician. This tool can be used in both inpatient and outpatient settings to reproducibly rate common signs and symptoms of opiate withdrawal and monitor these symptoms over time. The summed score for the complete scale can be used to help clinicians determine the stage or severity of opiate withdrawal and assess the level of physical dependence on opioids. Practitioners sometimes express concern about the objectivity of the items in the COWS; however, the symptoms of opioid withdrawal have been likened to a severe influenza infection (eg, nausea, vomiting, sweating, joint aches, agitation, tremor), and patients should not exceed the lowest score in most categories without exhibiting some observable sign or symptom of withdrawal.*

For each item, circle the number that best describes the patient's signs or symptom. Rate on just the apparent relationship to opiate withdrawal. For example, if heart rate is increased because the patient was jogging just prior to assessment, the increased pulse rate would not add to the score.

Patient: _____

Date: _____ Time: _____ (24 hour clock, midnight = 00:00)

Reason for this assessment: _____

Resting Pulse Rate: _____ beats/minute
Measured after patient is sitting or lying for one minute
  0 pulse rate 80 or below
  1 pulse rate 81–100
  2 pulse rate 101–120
  4 pulse rate greater than 120

Sweating: over past 1/2 hour not accounted for by room temperature or patient activity
  0 no report of chills or flushing
  1 subjective report of chills or flushing
  2 flushed or observable moistness on face

  3 beads of sweat on brow or face
  4 sweat streaming off face

Restlessness: observation during assessment
  0 able to sit still
  1 reports difficulty sitting still, but is able to do so
  3 frequent shifting or extraneous movements of legs/arms
  5 unable to sit still for more than a few seconds

Pupil Size
  0 pupils pinned or normal size for room light
  1 pupils possibly larger than normal for room light
  2 pupils moderately dilated
  5 pupils so dilated that only the rim of the iris is visible

Bone or Joint Aches: if patient was having pain previously, only the additional component attributed to opiate withdrawal is scored
  0 not present
  1 mild diffuse discomfort
  2 patient reports severe diffuse aching of joints/muscles
  4 patient is rubbing joints or muscles and is unable to sit still because of discomfort

Runny Nose or Tearing: not accounted for by cold symptoms or allergies
  0 not present
  1 nasal stuffiness or unusually moist eyes
  2 nose running or tearing
  4 nose constantly running or tears streaming down cheeks

GI Upset: over last 1/2 hour
  0 no GI symptoms
  1 stomach cramps
  2 nausea or loose stool
  3 vomiting or diarrhea
  5 multiple episodes of diarrhea or vomiting

Tremor: observation of outstretched hands
  0 no tremor
  1 tremor can be felt, but not observed
  2 slight tremor observable
  4 gross tremor or muscle twitching

Yawning: observation during assessment

   0 no yawning

   1 yawning once or twice during assessment

   2 yawning three or more times during assessment

   4 yawning several times/minute

Anxiety or Irritability

   0 none

   1 patient reports increasing irritability or anxiousness

   2 patient obviously irritable or anxious

   4 patient so irritable or anxious that participation in the assessment is difficult

Gooseflesh Skin

   0 skin is smooth

   3 piloerection of skin can be felt or hairs standing up on arms

   5 prominent piloerection

Total Score _____

The total score is the sum of all 11 items

Initials of person completing assessment:_____

Score: 5–12 = mild; 13–24 = moderate; 25–36 = moderately severe; more than 36 = severe withdrawal.

This version may be copied and used clinically.

Source: Wesson, D. R., & Ling, W. (2003). The Clinical Opiate Withdrawal Scale (COWS). *J Psychoactive Drugs*, 35(2), 253–259.

DRUG USE QUESTIONNAIRE (DAST-10)

AUTHOR'S NOTE: *The **DAST** is a screening tool that can be given to patients to complete in the waiting room. A higher score is not a diagnosis of a substance use disorder—it informs the clinician that there is a higher likelihood of a diagnosis, so it is worthwhile to proceed with gathering more information to make a diagnosis.*

Name: _____ Date: _____

The following questions concern information about your potential involvement with drugs excluding alcohol and tobacco during the past 12 months. Carefully read each question and decide if your answer is "YES" or "NO". Then, check the appropriate box beside the question.

When the words "drug abuse" are used, they mean the use of prescribed or over-the-counter medications used in excess of the directions and any non-medical use of any drugs. The various classes of drugs may include but are not limited to: cannabis (eg, marijuana, hash), solvents (eg, gas, paints, etc), tranquilizers (eg, Valium), barbiturates, cocaine, and stimulants (eg, speed), hallucinogens (eg, LSD), or narcotics (eg, heroin). Remember that the questions do not include alcohol or tobacco.

Please answer every question. If you have difficulty with a question then choose the response that is mostly right.

These questions refer to the past 12 months only.	YES	NO
1. Have you used drugs other than those required for medical reasons?		
2. Do you abuse more than one drug at a time?		
3. Are you always able to stop using drugs when you want to?		
4. Have you had "blackouts" or "flashbacks" as a result of drug use?		
5. Do you ever feel bad or guilty about your drug use?		
6. Does your spouse (or parent) ever complain about your involvement with drugs?		
7. Have you neglected your family because of your use of drugs?		
8. Have you engaged in illegal activities in order to obtain drugs?		

9.	Have you ever experienced withdrawal symptoms (felt sick) when you stopped taking drugs?		
10.	Have you had medical problems as a result of your drug use (eg, memory loss, hepatitis, convulsions, bleeding, etc)?		
DAST Score			
* See scoring instructions for correct scoring procedures			

Drug Use Questionnaire (DAST-10)
Administration & Interpretation

Instructions

The DAST-10 is a 10-item, yes/no, self-report instrument that has been shortened from the 28-item DAST and should take less than 8 minutes to complete. The DAST-10 was designed to provide a brief instrument for clinical screening and treatment evaluation and can be used with adults and older youth. It is **strongly recommended** that the SMAST be used along with the DAST-10 unless there is a clear indication that the client uses NO ALCOHOL at all. The answer options for each item are "YES" or "NO". The DAST-10 is a self-administered screening instrument.

Scoring and Interpretation—For the DAST-10, score 1 point for each question answered "YES", except for question (3) for which a "NO" answer receives 1 point and a "YES" answer receives 0 points. Add up the points and interpret as follows:

DAST-10 Score	Degree of Problem Related to Drug Abuse	Suggested Action
0	No problems reported	None at this time.
1–2	Low level	Monitor, reassess at a later date.
3–5	Moderate level	Further investigation is required.
6–8	Substantial level	Assessment required.
9–10	Severe level	Assessment required.

FAGERSTRÖM TEST FOR NICOTINE DEPENDENCE

AUTHOR'S NOTE: *The Fagerström Test for Nicotine Dependence helps determine the severity of physical dependence on nicotine. It asks about tobacco use in specific situations instead of symptoms of withdrawal. Higher scores mean higher need for nicotine replacement therapy or more support for smoking cessation. It can be applied to use of e-cigarettes or smokeless tobacco (chew, snuff) as well.*

PLEASE SELECT FOR EACH QUESTION		
How soon after waking do you smoke your first cigarette?	Within 5 minutes 5–30 minutes	____ 3 ____ 2
Do you find it difficult to refrain from smoking in places where it is forbidden? eg, church, library, etc.	Yes No	____ 1 ____ 0
Which cigarette would you hate to give up?	The first in the morning Any other	____ 1 ____ 0
How many cigarettes a day do you smoke?	10 or less 11–20 21–30	____ 0 ____ 1 ____ 2
Do you smoke more frequently in the morning?	Yes No	____ 1 ____ 0
Do you smoke even if you are sick in bed most of the day?	Yes No	____ 1 ____ 0
Total Score		
SCORE _____ 1–2 = low dependence; 3–4 = low to moderate dependence; 5–7 = moderate dependence; 8+ = high dependence		

Source: Heatherton et al, *Br J Addict* 1991;86:1119–1127.

Add up the scores from the questionnaire.

Score of 1–2: Patients who score between 1 and 2 are classified as having a low dependence on nicotine. This suggests that they may not need nicotine replacement therapy (NRT), although it is recommended that they still be monitored for withdrawal symptoms.

Score of 3–4: Patients who score 3 or 4 are considered to have a low to moderate dependence on nicotine and can be offered patches, inhaler, lozenges, or gum.

Score of 5–7: Patients who score 5–7 are considered moderately dependent on nicotine and can be offered patches, inhaler, lozenges, or gum. They can also be offered the combined therapy of patches with lozenges and gum.

Score of 8 and over: Patients who score 8 and over are considered highly dependent on nicotine and can be offered patches, inhaler, lozenges, and/or gum. They can also be offered the combined therapy of patches and lozenges or gum.

RECOMMENDED READING

Here are just a few of the resources that I have found to be helpful. I think you will find them informative.

Books

Miller S, Fiellin D, Saitz R, eds. *Principles of Addiction Medicine.* 6th ed. Chevy Chase, MD: American Society of Addiction Medicine, Inc.; 2017

Miller WR and Rollnick S. *Motivational Interviewing: Helping People Change.* 3rd ed. New York: The Guilford Press; 2013

Center for Substance Abuse Treatment. *Substance Abuse Treatment for Persons With Co-Occurring Disorders.* Treatment Improvement Protocol (TIP) Series No. 42. HHS Publication No. (SMA) 13-3992. Rockville, MD: Substance Abuse and Mental Health Services Administration; 2005

Articles

Leshner AI. Addiction is a brain disease. *Issues in Science and Technology* 2001;17:75–80

Weaver MF, Jarvis MAE, Schnoll SH. Role of the primary care physician in problems of substance abuse. *Archives of Internal Medicine* 1999;159(9):913–924

Websites

www.drugabuse.gov (National Institute on Drug Abuse)

www.pcssmat.org (Providers' Clinical Support System for Medication-Assisted Treatment)

www.aa.org (Alcoholics Anonymous)

www.erowid.org (Erowid Center for information about psychoactive chemicals)

www.dancesafe.org (harm reduction organization targeted at the electronic music community)

REFERENCES

Bien, T. H., Miller, W. R., & Tonigan, J. S. (1993). Brief interventions for alcohol problems: A review. *Addiction, 88*(3), 315–335.

Billioti de Gage, S., Pariente, A., & Bégaud, B. (2015). Is there really a link between benzodiazepine use and the risk of dementia? *Expert Opin Drug Saf, 14*(5), 733–747. doi:10.1517/14740338.2015.1014796

Bradizza, C. M., Stasiewicz, P. R., & Paas, N. D. (2006). Relapse to alcohol and drug use among individuals diagnosed with co-occurring mental health and substance use disorders: A review. *Clinical Psychology Review, 26*(2), 162–178.

Capriola, M. (2013). Synthetic cathinone abuse. *Clin Pharmacol, 5*(1), 109–115. doi:10.2147/CPAA.S42832

Cheever, S. (1999). The healer: Bill W. *Time, 153*(23), 201–204.

Compton, W. M., Thomas, Y. F., Stinson F. S., et al. (2007). Prevalence, correlates, disability, and comorbidity of DSM-IV drug abuse and dependence in the United States: Results from the national epidemiologic survey on alcohol and related conditions. *Arch Gen Psychiatry, 64*(5), 566–576.

Ebbert, J. O., Hughes, J. R., West, R. J., et al. (2015). Effect of varenicline on smoking cessation through smoking reduction: A randomized clinical trial. *JAMA, 313*(7), 687–694. doi:10.1001/jama.2015.280

Ferri, M., Amato, L., & Davoli, M. (2006). Alcoholics Anonymous and other 12-step programmes for alcohol dependence. *Cochrane Database Syst Rev, 2006* Jul 19, CD005032.

Gage, S. H., Jones, H. J., Burgess, S., et al. (2016). Assessing causality in associations between cannabis use and schizophrenia risk: A two-sample Mendelian randomization study. *Psychol Med, 2016* Dec 8, 1–10 [Epub ahead of print].

Gao, K., Sheehan, D. V., & Calabrese, J. R. (2009). Atypical antipsychotics in primary generalized anxiety disorder or comorbid with mood disorders. *Expert Rev Neurother, 9*(8), 1147–1158. doi:10.1586/ern.09.37

Gommoll, C., Durgam, S., Mathews, M., et al. (2015). A double-blind, randomized, placebo-controlled, fixed-dose phase III study of vilazodone in patients with generalized anxiety disorder. *Depress Anxiety, 32*(6), 451–459. doi:10.1002/da.22365

Gouzoulis-Mayfrank, E., Daumann, J., Tuchtenhagen, F., et al. (2000). Impaired cognitive performance in drug free users of recreational ecstasy (MDMA). *J Neurol Neurosurg and Psychiatry, 68*(6), 719–725. doi:10.1136/jnnp.68.6.719

Hasin, D. S., Stinson, F. S., Ogburn, E., et al. (2007). Prevalence, correlates, disability, and comorbidity of DSM-IV alcohol abuse and dependence in the

United States: Results from the National Epidemiologic Survey on Alcohol and Related Conditions. *Arch Gen Psychiatry, 64*(7), 830–842.

Hurt, R. D., Sachs, D. P. L., Glover, E. D., et al. (1997). A comparison of sustained-release bupropion and placebo for smoking cessation. *NEJM, 337*(17), 1195–1202. doi:10.1056/NEJM199710233371703

Jones, H. E., Johnson, R. E., Jasinski, D. R., et al. (2005). Buprenorphine versus methadone in the treatment of pregnant opioid-dependent patients: Effects on the neonatal abstinence syndrome. *Drug Alcohol Depend, 79*(1), 1–10.

Jones, H. E., Kaltenbach, K., Heil, S. H., et al. (2010). Neonatal abstinence syndrome after methadone or buprenorphine exposure. *N Engl J Med, 363*, 2320–2331. doi:10.1056/NEJMoa1005359

Kaskutas, L. A. (2009). Alcoholics Anonymous effectiveness: Faith meets science. *J Addict Dis, 28*(2), 145–157. doi:10.1080/10550880902772464

Krentzman, A. R., Cranford, J. A., & Robinson, E. A. (2013). Multiple dimensions of spirituality in recovery: A lagged mediational analysis of Alcoholics Anonymous' principal theoretical mechanism of behavior change. *Substance Abuse, 34*(1), 20–32. doi:10.1080/08897077.2012.691449

Kushner, M. G., Donahue, C., Sletten, S., et al. (2006). Cognitive behavioral treatment of comorbid anxiety disorder in alcoholism treatment patients: Presentation of a prototype program and future directions. *J Mental Health, 15*(6), 697–707. doi:10.1080/09638230600998946

Levin, F. R., Mariani, J. J., Brooks, D. J., et al. (2011). Dronabinol for the treatment of cannabis dependence: A randomized, double-blind, placebo-controlled trial. *Drug and Alcohol Dependence, 116*(1–3), 142–150. doi:10.1016/j.drugalcdep.2010.12.010

Ligresti, A., De Petrocellis, L., & Di Marzo, V. (2016). From phytocannabinoids to cannabinoid receptors and endocannabinoids: Pleiotropic physiological and pathological roles through complex pharmacology. *Physiol Rev, 96*(4), 1593–1659. doi:10.1152/physrev.00002.2016

Lingford-Hughes, A., Potokar, J., & Nutt, D. (2002). Treating anxiety complicated by substance misuse. *Adv Psychiatr Treat, 8*(2), 107–116. doi:10.1192/apt.8.2.107

Llorca, P. M., Spadone, C., Sol, O., et al. (2002). Efficacy and safety of hydroxyzine in the treatment of generalized anxiety disorder: A 3-month double-blind study. *J Clin Psychiatry, 63*(11), 1020–1027.

Lubman, D. I., Cheetham, A., & Yücel, M. (2015). Cannabis and adolescent brain development. *Pharmacol Ther, 148*, 1–16. doi:10.1016/j.pharmthera.2014.11.009

Lussier, J. P., Heil, S. H., Mongeon, J. A., et al. (2006). A meta-analysis of voucher-based reinforcement therapy for substance use disorders. *Addiction, 101*(2), 192–203.

Martin, P. R., Adinoff, B., Weingartner, H., et al. (1986). Alcoholic organic brain disease: Nosology and pathophysiologic mechanisms. *Prog Neuropsychopharmacol Biol Psychiatry, 10*(2), 147–164.

Martinotti, G., Di Nicola, M., Tedeschi, D., et al. (2010). Pregabalin versus naltrexone in alcohol dependence: A randomised, double-blind, comparison trial. *J Psychopharmacol, 24*(9), 1367–1374. doi:10.1177/0269881109102623

McKay, J. R., Lynch, K. G., Coviello, D., et al. (2010). Randomized trial of continuing care enhancements for cocaine-dependent patients following initial engagement. *J Consult Clin Psychol, 78*(1), 111–120. doi:10.1037/a0018139

Myrick, H., Malcolm, R., Randall, P. K., et al. (2009). A double-blind trial of gabapentin versus lorazepam in the treatment of alcohol withdrawal. *Alcohol Clin Exp Res, 33*(9), 1582–1588. doi:10.1111/j.1530-0277.2009.00986.x

Nunes, E. V., & Levin, F. R. (2004). Treatment of depression in patients with alcohol or other drug dependence: A meta-analysis. *JAMA, 291*(15), 1887–1996.

Pande, A. C., Davidson, J. R., Jefferson, J. W., et al. (1999). Treatment of social phobia with gabapentin: A placebo-controlled study. *J Clin Psychopharmacol, 19*(4), 341–348.

Pi-Sunyer, F. X., Aronne, L. J., Heshmati, H. M., et al. (2006). Effect of rimonabant, a cannabinoid-1 receptor blocker, on weight and cardiometabolic risk factors in overweight or obese patients: RIO-North America: A randomized controlled trial. *JAMA, 295*(7), 761–775.

Project MATCH Research Group. (1997). Matching alcoholism treatments to client heterogeneity: Project MATCH posttreatment drinking outcomes. *J Stud Alcohol, 58*(1), 7–29.

Regier, D. A., Farmer, M. E., Rae, D. S., et al. (1990). Comorbidity of mental disorders with alcohol and other drug abuse. Results from the Epidemiologic Catchment Area (ECA) Study. *JAMA, 264*(19), 2511–2518.

Reinhold, J. A., & Rickels, K. (2015). Pharmacological treatment for generalized anxiety disorder in adults: An update. *Expert Opin Pharmacother, 16*(11), 1669–1681. doi:10.1517/14656566.2015.1059424

Sansone, R. A., & Sansone, L. A. (2010). Is seroquel developing an illicit reputation for misuse/abuse? *Psychiatry (Edgmont), 7*(1), 13–16.

Sechi, G., & Serra, A. (2007). Wernicke's encephalopathy: New clinical settings and recent advances in diagnosis and management. *Lancet Neurol, 6*(5), 442–455.

Smith, P. C., Schmidt, S. M., Allensworth-Davies, D., et al. (2009). Primary care validation of a single-question alcohol screening test. *J Gen Intern Med, 24*(7), 783–788. doi:10.1007/s11606-009-0928-6

Suzuki, J., Poklis, J. L., & Poklis, A. (2014). "My friend said it was good LSD": A suicide attempt following analytically confirmed 25I-NBOMe ingestion.

Journal of Psychoactive Drugs, 46(5), 379–382. doi:10.1080/02791072.2014 .960111

Thomas, K. H., Martin, R. M., Knipe, D. W., et al. (2015). Risk of neuropsychiatric adverse events associated with varenicline: Systematic review and meta-analysis. *BMJ, 350,* h1109. doi:10.1136/bmj.h1109

Thomson, A. D., Cook, C. C. H., Touquet, R., et al. (2002). The Royal College of Physicians report on alcohol: Guidelines for managing Wernicke's encephalopathy in the accident and emergency department. *Alcohol and Alcoholism, 37*(6), 513–521. doi:10.1093/alcalc/37.6.513

Timko, C., Halvorson, M., Kong, C., et al. (2015). Social processes explaining the benefits of Al-Anon participation. *Psychol Addict Behav, 29*(4), 856–863. doi:10.1037/adb0000067

Tonigan, J. S., Connors, G. J., & Miller, W. R. (2003). Participation and involvement in Alcoholics Anonymous. In T. F. Babor & F. K. Del Boca (Eds.), *Treatment Matching in Alcoholism* (184–204). New York: Cambridge University Press.

Tupper, K. W., Wood, E., Yensen, R., et al. (2015). Psychedelic medicine: A re-emerging therapeutic paradigm. *CMAJ, 187*(14), 1054–1059. doi:10.1503/ cmaj.141124

Weaver, M. F. (2013). Choices for patients and clinicians: Ethics and legal issues. In R. Saitz (Ed.), *Addressing Unhealthy Alcohol Use in Primary Care* (195–205). New York: Springer.

Weaver, M. F., Hopper, J. A., & Gunderson, E. W. (2015). Designer drugs 2015: Assessment and management. *Addict Sci Clin Pract, 10*(1), 8. doi:10.1186/ s13722-015-0024-7

Yu, C., & McClellan, J. (2016). Genetics of substance use disorders. *Child Adolesc Psychiatr Clin N Am, 25*(3), 377–385. doi:10.1016/j.chc.2016.02.002

Zhong, G., Wang, Y., Zhang, Y., et al. (2015). Association between benzodiazepine use and dementia: A meta-analysis. *PLoS ONE, 10*(5), e0127836. doi:10.1371/ journal.pone.0127836

SELF-TEST ANSWER KEY

If you purchased CME credit with this book, your CME post-test can be accessed when you are logged in at www.thecarlatreport.com/ AddictionGuide. Please keep in mind that the question and answer order for that CME post-test are different than what you see in these self-test study questions.

Chapter 1:
1. a
2. d
3. a

Chapter 2:
1. b
2. c
3. d

Chapter 3:
1. c
2. d
3. c

Chapter 4:
1. b
2. d
3. c

Chapter 5:
1. d
2. c
3. a

Chapter 6:
1. d
2. b
3. d

Chapter 7:
1. d
2. c
3. c

Chapter 8:
1. a
2. c
3. a

Chapter 9:
1. c
2. b
3. c

Chapter 10:
1. a
2. b
3. c

Chapter 11:
1. c
2. b
3. a

Chapter 12:
1. c
2. b
3. d

Chapter 13:
1. c
2. d
3. a

Chapter 14:
1. d
2. a
3. b

Index

Note: Page numbers followed by *f* indicate figures; *t* indicates tables.

A

Acamprostate (Campral), for alcoholism, 112–113, 112t
Addiction
  genetics of, 3–4
  neurobiology of, 2–3
Addiction counselors and therapists, 36–37
Addiction services, 35–45
Addiction treatment programs, 39–44, 39t
  court-mandated programs, 43–44
  holding beds, 39t, 43
  intensive outpatient programs (IOP), 39t, 40
  long-term residential, 39t, 42
  partial hospital programs (PHP), 39t, 40–41
  residential rehab, 39t, 41
  sober houses, 39t, 42
ADHD stimulants, 187–188
Al-Anon, 77–79
Alcohol, 93–116
  assessing consumption, 99–100
  CDC definitions of a standard drink, 100
  drug screens and, 98
  essentials of, 94
  immediate effects, 94–95
  long-term effects, 95
  screening question, 7
  withdrawal syndrome, 97–98
Alcoholics Anonymous (AA), 63–80. *see also* Twelve-Step programs
  alternatives, 77–78
  The Big book, 66
  history of, 64
  list of steps, 67–70, 78
  potential barriers to attendance, 76–77
  sponsorship, 73
  Twelve Traditions, 70–71
Alcohol use disorder
  assessment, 98–103
  common medical complications of, 96t

detox, 105–109
DSM-5 criteria, 101–103
DSM-focused questions, 102
medication-assisted treatment, 109–114
planning treatment strategy, 104
treatment, 103–114
Alprazolam (Xanax), 117
  characteristics of, 125t
American Academy of Addiction Psychiatry, 38
American Society of Addiction Medicine, criteria, 37
Amphetamines, false positives, 27t
Amyl nitrite, 213
Angel dust, 207t, 211
Antianxiety medications, 86t
Anxiety disorders, substance use and, 85

B

Barbiturates, 117–127
  false positives, 27t
Bath salts, 198–200
Benzodiazepines, 117–127
  false positives, 27t, 28
  for substance-abusing patients, 87
Bipolar disorder, substance use and, 83–84
Blood testing, 22
Breath testing, 23
Brief intervention, 53
Buprenorphine, 160t
  different formulations, 174–177, 176t
  maintenance *versus* tapering, 173–174
  treatment of opioid abuse, 169–177
  typical causes of failure, 174
Buprenorphine/naloxone, 160t
  treatment of opioid abuse, 170
Bupropion (Wellbutrin, Zyban), tobacco cessation drug, 138–139, 139t
Buspirone, for substance-abusing patients, 86t, 88
Butyl nitrite, 213

C

Caffeine
  screening question, 7
  as stimulants, 188
CAGE questionnaire, 99
Cannabinoids, synthetic, 196–198
Cannabis, 145–156
  assessment, 150–151
  behavioral treatment, 154
  brain development and, 154
  edibles, 149–150
  hash oils, 149, 149t
  hyperemesis syndrome, 150
  immediate effects, 146
  long-term effects, 146–147
  medications, 153–154
  motivational interviewing, 151–153
  physical effects, 147–148
  screening question, 8
  smoked products, 148–149, 149t
  synthetic cannabinoids, 150
  treatment, 151–153
  withdrawal, 148
Carbamazepine (Tegretol), for alcohol
    detox, 109
Carisoprodol (Soma), 119
Celebrate Recovery, 77
Chlordiazepoxide (Librium), 117
  characteristics of, 125t
  outpatient alcohol detox, 106
Chronic cannabis syndrome, 147. see also
    Cannabis
Clinical Institute Withdrawal Assessment
    of Alcohol Scale, Revised
    (CIWA-AR), 105–109217–220
Clinical Opiate Withdrawal Scale (COWS),
    221–223
Clonazepam (Klonopin)
  characteristics of, 125t
  outpatient alcohol detox, 106
Clonidine
  tobacco cessation, 139t
  use in alcohol detox, 109
  use in opioid withdrawal, 169t
Club drugs, 209–210
Cocaine, false positives, 27t
Cocaine (Roxane), 185–187, 186t

Codeine, 158, 160t
Cognitive behavioral therapy (CBT), 48
  Project MATCH, 65–67
Cold turkey, origins of the term, 162
Confirmatory testing (CT), 26
Contingency management programs, use in
    cocaine abuse, 191–192
Court-mandated programs, 43–44

D

Dementia and brain disorders, alcoholism
    and, 96t
Denial, opioid use disorder, 165
Department of Transportation (DOT),
    protocol for urine collection, 24–26
Depression, substance use and, 84–85
Desensitization, 2–3
Designer drugs, 195–202, 201t
  screening question, 9
Detox, 39–40, 39t. see also Inpatient detox;
    Outpatient detox
  alcohol, 105–109
  methadone maintenance and, 178
  opioids, 167–169
  sedatives, 122–124
Dextroamphetamine (Adderall), 186t
Diazepam (Valium), 117
  characteristics of, 125t
Dimethyltryptamine (DMT), 207t, 208
Dissociative anesthetics, 211–212
Disulfiram (Antabuse), 113–114, 113t
Dopamine (DA), 2–3
Drano or laundry bleach, false negatives,
    29t
Dronabinol (Marinol), 147
Drug testing
  broaching the issue, 18–19
  collecting the sample, 23–26
  discussing problematic results, 30–31
  disputing results, 31–32
  false testing, 28–30, 29t
  false positives, 27–28, 27t
  frequency of, 32–33
  medical review officer, 32
  results, 26–32
  types, 20–23, 20t
  when to order a drug screen, 18

Drug Use Questionnaire (DAST-10), 224–225
DSM-5 criteria
  alcohol use disorder, 101–103
  mnemonic for substance use disorder, 11
  nicotine use disorder, 132–134
  opioid use disorder, 162
  sedative use disorder, 121
  substance use disorder, 9–13, 12*f*
Dual diagnosis, 81–92

E

Ecstasy (MDMA), 196, 210–215
Electronic cigarettes, 131–132

F

Fagerström Test for Nicotine Dependence, 133, 226–227
False negatives, 28–30
False positives, 27, 27*t*
Fentanyl, 158, 160*t*
Flunitrazepam (Rohypnol), 207*t*, 213
FRAMES technique, 53

G

GABA-A receptors
  alcohol use disorder and, 4, 94
  medications for modulation, 86*t*
Gabapentin (Neurontin)
  for alcohol detox, 109
  for substance-abusing patients, 86*t*, 89
Gamma hydroxybutyrate (GHB), 212
Gastrointestinal issues, alcoholism and, 96*t*
Generalized anxiety disorder (GAD), 82
Glutaraldehyde, false negatives, 29*t*
Gorski, Terence, advice on relapse prevention, 58–59

H

Hair testing, 22
Halfway house. *see* Sober house
Hallucinogens, 206–210, 207*t*
  assessment, 214
  screening question, 9
  synthetic, 200–202
  treatment, 209, 214

HALT reminder, 55
Hash oils, 149, 149*t*
Herbal medications. *see* Natural medications
Heroin, 158, 160*t*
Holding beds, 39*t*, 43
Hydrocodone, 158, 160*t*
Hydrogen peroxide, false negatives, 29*t*
Hydromorphone, 160*t*
Hydroxyzine (Atarax, Vistaril), for substance-abusing patients, 86*t*, 88
Hyperemesis syndrome, 150

I

Ibuprofen, use in opioid withdrawal, 169*t*
Inhalants, 213–214
  screening question, 9
Insurance billing, substance abuse counseling, 51
Intensive outpatient programs (IOP), 39*t*, 40
Interventionists, 38

J

Journaling, relapse avoidance, 59

K

K2, 196
Ketamine, 196, 207*t*, 212
Kicking the habit, origins of the term, 162

L

Liquid hand soap, false negatives, 29*t*
Liver disease, alcoholism and, 96*t*
Long-term residential programs, 39*t*, 42
Loperamide, use in opioid withdrawal, 169*t*
Lorazepam (Ativan)
  characteristics of, 125*t*
  outpatient alcohol detox, 106
Lysergic acid diethylamide (LSD), 206–207, 207*t*

M

Medical review officer (MRO), 32
Meperidine, 160*t*
Mephedrone, 198

Mescaline, 207t, 208
  derivatives, 209
Methadone, 158, 160t
Methadone maintenance
  detox problems, 178
  how to dose, 178–179
  opioid abuse, 177–181
Methamphetamine (Desoxyn), 186t, 187,
    207t
Methlphenidate (Ritalin, Concerta), 186t
Methylenedioxy-amphetamine (MDA),
    207t
Methylenedioxy-methamphetamine
    (MDMA, ecstasy), 207t, 210–215
Methylone, 198
Metoclopramide, use in alcohol detox, 109
Morphine, 158, 160t
Motivational enhancement therapy
    (MET), Project MATCH, 65–67
Motivational interviewing (MI), 48–53
  brief intervention with, 53
  cannabis, 151–153
  opioid use disorder, 163–165
  stages of change, 48–52, 49t

N

Nail testing, 23
Naloxone, 180–181
Naltrexone (Revia; Vivitrol), for
    alcoholism, 109–112, 109t, 111t
Nar-Anon, 77–79
Narcotics Anonymous (NA), 63–80
Natural medications (valerian), for
    substance-abusing patients, 86t,
    89–90
N-bomb, 200
251-NBOMe, 200
Neurocognitive disorders, substance use
    and, 86
Nicotine, 129–143
  electronic cigarettes, 131–132
  immediate effects, 130–131
  long-term effects, 131
  screening question, 7
  withdrawal syndrome, 131
Nicotine replacement therapy (NRT),
    135–137
  combination, 137

  lozenge, 137, 137t
  patch, 136, 137t
  spray, 137, 137t
Nitric oxide, 213
Nitrous oxide, 213
Nonalcoholic beers, 57
Nortriptyline, tobacco cessation, 139t

O

Opioid overdose, naloxone and, 180–181
Opioids
  false positives, 27, 27t
  screening question, 9
Opioid use disorder, 157–183
  assessment, 162–167
  buprenorphine, 169–176
  commonly used drugs, 160t
  DSM-5 criteria, 162
  long-term effects, 161
  medical issues and labs, 166–167
  methadone maintenance treatment,
    177–181
  motivational interviewing, 163–165
  physical effects, 159–160
  psychosocial interventions, 181
  sexual function, 159
  treatment, 167–181
  vivitrol treatment, 179–180
  withdrawal, 161
Outpatient detox
  alcohol, 106–108
  opioids, 168–169
Outpatient tapering, opioids, 167–168
  medications for withdrawal symptoms,
    169t
  switching to different opioid, 168
Oxazepam (Serax)
  characteristics of, 125t
  outpatient alcohol detox, 106
Oxycodone, 160t
Oxymorphone, 160t

P

Partial hospital programs (PHP), 39t,
    40–41
Peripheral neuropathy, alcoholism and, 96t
pH, normal urine, 25

Phencyclidine (PCP), 207t, 211
  false positives, 27t, 28
Phenobarbital
  characteristics of, 125t
  outpatient alcohol detox, 106–107, 108t
  outpatient sedative detox, 122–124
Potassium nitrite (Klear, Whizzies), false
      negatives, 29t
Pregabalin (Lyrica), for substance-abusing
      patients, 86t, 88
Prochlorperazine, use in opioid withdrawal,
      169t
Project MATCH, 65–67
Psilocybin, 207t, 208
Psychotherapy, 47–61
Psychotic disorders, substance use and, 85
Pyridinum chlorochromate (Urine Luck),
      false negatives, 29t

Q

Quetiapine (Seroquel), for substance-
      abusing patients, 86t, 89

R

Relapse
  common causes, 55–58
  journaling for, 59
  tobacco use, 140–141
Relapse prevention therapy (RPT), 54–59
Residential rehab, 39t, 41

S

Saliva testing, 22
SAMHSA treatment locator, 38
Sample collection, 23–26
Secobarbital (Seconal), 119
Secular Organization for Sobriety (SOS),
      77
Sedatives, 117–127
  characteristics of, 125t
  club, 212–213
  immediate effects, 118
  long-term effects, 119–120
Sedative use disorder
  assessment, 120–121
  detox, 122–124
  DSM-5 criteria for, 120–12121

relapse prevention, 124–125
  treatment, 121–122
Self-efficacy, 53
Self-medication, relapse and, 55–56
SMART Recovery, 77
SNRIs
  for substance-abusing patients, 86t, 87
  use for cannabis, 153–154
Sober houses, 39t, 42
Speaker meetings (AA), 72
Special K, 212
Specific gravity, normal urine, 25
Speedball overdoses, 189
Spice, 196–197
Sponsorship, how it works, 73
SSRIs, 82
  for substance-abusing patients, 86t, 87
  use for cannabis, 153–154
Stages of Change model, 49t
Stimulants, 185–194, 186t
  assessment, 190–191
  false positives, 28
  immediate effects, 188–189
  long-term effects, 190
  screening question, 9
  treatment, 191–192
  withdrawal, 190
Suboxone, 174
Substance use disorder
  assessment of, 4–10
  billing insurance companies, 51
  definition, 2–4
  DSM-5 criteria for, 9–16
  potential antianxiety medications for use
      in, 86t
  screening questions
    general, 5–7
    specific substances, 7–9
    specific psychiatric disorders with,
      83–86
Sweat testing, 22–23
Synthetic cannabinoids, 196–198, 201t
  assessment, 198
  treatment, 198
  withdrawal syndromes, 197
Synthetic cathinones, 198–200, 201t
  assessment and treatment, 199–200
  excited delirium, 200

psychiatric consequences, 200
withdrawal syndromes, 199
Synthetic hallucinogens, 200–202
assessment and treatment, 202
withdrawal syndromes, 202

T

Table salt, false negatives, 29t
Tetrahydrocannabinoid (THC), 145–156
THC, false positives, 27t
The Association for Addiction
Professionals (NAADAC), 36–37
Tobacco use disorder
assessment, 132–134
DSM-5 criteria, 132–134
non-pharmacologic treatment, 134–135
off-label meds, 139, 139t
pharmacologic treatment, 135–140
quitting and preventing relapse, 140–141
Tramadol, 158, 160t
Trazodone
use in alcohol detox, 109
use in opioid withdrawal, 169t
Twelve step facilitation (TSF), Project
MATCH, 65–67
Twelve-step program, 39, 39t, 63–80. see
also Alcoholics Anonymous (AA)
list of steps, 67–70, 75–76, 78

U

Urine testing, 20–22, 21t
best practices for collection, 24–26
cheating, 23–24

lab analysis and confirmatory testing, 26
point-of-care (POC), 26
preliminary dipstick, 25
timing of, 25–26

V

Varenicline (Chantix), tobacco cessation
drug, 137–138, 138t
Vinegar, false negatives, 29t
Visine OTC eye drops, false negatives, 29t
Vivitrol, opioid use disorder, 179–180

W

Whizzinator, 24
Wilson, Bill (AA), 64
Withdrawal syndromes, 3
alcohol, 97–98
cannabis, 148
nicotine, 131
opioids, 161–162, 169t
stimulants, 190
synthetic cannabinoids, 197
synthetic hallucinogens, 202

X

Xanax, street names, 124

Z

Zaleplon (Sonata), characteristics of, 125t
Z-drugs. see Benzodiazepines
Zolpidem (Ambien or Intermezzo), 117,
125t

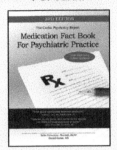
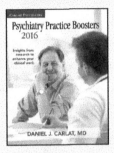
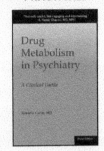
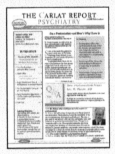
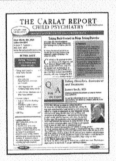